EVIDENCE-BASED HEALTHCARE IN CONTEXT

For Suvena

Evidence-Based Healthcare in Context

Critical Social Science Perspectives

Edited by

ALEX BROOM
University of Queensland, Australia
and

JON ADAMS
University of Technology, Sydney, Australia

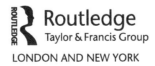

LONDON AND NEW YORK

First published 2012 by Ashgate Publishing

Published 2016 by Routledge
2 Park Square, Milton Park, Abingdon, Oxfordshire OX14 4RN
711 Third Avenue, New York, NY 10017, USA

First issued in paperback 2016

Routledge is an imprint of the Taylor & Francis Group, an informa business

British Library Cataloguing in Publication Data
Evidence-based healthcare in context : critical social
   science perspectives.
   1. Evidence-based medicine. 2. Medicine--Decision making.
   3. Social medicine.
   I. Broom, Alex. II. Adams, Jon, 1971-
   616'.001-dc23

Library of Congress Cataloging-in-Publication Data
Broom, Alex.
   Evidence-based healthcare in context : critical social science
perspectives / by Alex Broom and Jon Adams.
      p. cm.
   Includes bibliographical references and index.
   ISBN 978-0-7546-7981-3 (hbk) 1. Evidence-based
medicine. 2. Social medicine. I. Adams, Jon, 1971- II. Title. III. Title:
Evidence based health care in context.
   R723.7.B76 2011
   362.1--dc23

2011040154

ISBN 13: 978-1-138-27415-0 (pbk)
ISBN 13: 978-0-7546-7981-3 (hbk)

Contents

List of Contributors

Jon Adams is Professor of Public Health at the University of Technology Sydney and holds an NHMRC Career Development Fellowship in CAM and women's health. He is Executive Director of the Network of Researchers in the Public Health of Complementary and Alternative Medicine (www.norphcam.org) and a Senior Fellow of the International Brisbane Initiative, Department of Primary Health Care, University of Oxford. Recent titles include *The Mainstreaming of Complementary and Alternative Medicine: Studies in Social Context* (Routledge), *Complementary and Alternative Medicine in Nursing and Midwifery: Towards a Critical Social Science* (Routledge), *Researching Complementary and Alternative Medicine* (Routledge), and *Complementary and Integrative Medicine in Primary Health Care* (Imperial College Press).

Berit Brattheim is a Doctoral candidate within the field of Medical Technology, Faculty of Medicine, Norwegian University of Science and Technology (NTNU). Her PhD project centers on healthcare information systems, in particular an ethnographic investigation to explore the needs for process support in clinical practice. She is an Assistant Professor at the Department of Radiography, Sør-Trøndelag University College.

Alex Broom is Associate Professor of Sociology and Australia Research Council Future Fellow at the School of Social Science, the University of Queensland, Australia. He specialises in the sociology of traditional, complementary and alternative medicine (TCAM) and the sociology of cancer and end-of-life care, leading studies in Australia, the UK, Brazil, India, Pakistan and Sri Lanka. Alex is currently leading a cross-cultural comparative study of medical pluralism in Australia, India and Brazil, and a longitudinal qualitative study of end-of-life care in Australia. Recent co-authored and co-edited books include: *Traditional, Complementary and Alternative Medicine and Cancer Care* (Routledge, 2007), *Therapeutic Pluralism* (Routledge, 2008), *Men's Health: Body, Identity and Social Context* (Wiley-Blackwell, 2009), *Health, Culture and Religion in South Asia* (Routledge, 2011) and *Complementary and Integrative Medicine in Primary Health Care* (Imperial College Press, forthcoming). He is a Visiting Professor at Jawaharlal Nehru University (India) and Brunel University (London), and he is an Honorary Associate Professor at the University of Sydney (Australia).

Kevin Dew is Professor of Sociology at Victoria University of Wellington. In 2007 he was awarded the inaugural scholarship award from the Sociological

Association of Aotearoa/New Zealand for contributions to New Zealand Sociology. He is a founding member of the Applied Research on Communication in Health (ARCH) group. Current research activities include studies of interactions between health professionals and patients, and the social meanings of medications, which are supported by research grants from the Health Research Council and the Marsden Fund. He is on the international advisory boards of *Sociology of Health and Illness* and *Critical Public Health*, on the editorial boards of *The Australian and New Zealand Journal of Public Health* and *New Zealand Sociology*. His books include *The Cult and Science of Public Health: A Sociological Investigation, Borderland Practices: Regulating Alternative Therapy in New Zealand, Sociology of Health in New Zealand* (with Allison Kirkman), *Health Inequalities in Aotearoa New Zealand* (edited with Anna Matheson), *Health and Society in Aotearoa New Zealand* (edited with Peter Davis) and *Challenging Science: Issues for New Zealand Society in the 21st Century* (edited with Ruth Fitzgerald).

Rob Flynn, until his retirement in October 2011, was Professor of Sociology in the Centre for Social Research, School of Humanities, Languages and Social Sciences at the University of Salford, UK. He has researched and published widely about health services management and the regulation of medical professionals. Most recently he has been investigating public perceptions of risk surrounding hydrogen energy technologies.

Joanne Greenhalgh is Principal Research Fellow in the School of Sociology and Social Policy at the University of Leeds, UK. Her research has applied a range of social research methods to the design and evaluation of patient-reported outcome measures, and their application in clinical practice, and she has published widely in this field.

Arild Faxvaag is Associate Professor in Rheumatology at Faculty of Medicine, Norwegian University of Science and Technology (NTNU), a practicing rheumatologist at St. Olavs hospital, Trondheim, and the leader of Norwegian Centre for electronic patient records research. His research centers on: development of high quality clinical databases for collection of data from patient cohorts with the purpose of clinical decision support; systems for quality development; evaluation of electronic medical record systems from the perspective of clinicians; and, clinical decision support systems.

Dave Holmes is Professor and University Research Chair in Forensic Nursing. He is also Director and Associate Dean, School of Nursing, Faculty of Health Sciences at the University of Ottawa, Canada. Most of his work, comments, essays, analyses and research are based on the poststructuralist works of Deleuze and Guattari, and Michel Foucault. His works have been published in top-tier journals in nursing, criminology, sociology and medicine. Professor Holmes has published over 110 articles in peer reviewed journals and 25 book chapters. He is co-editor of *Critical Interventions in the Ethics of Health Care* (Ashgate, 2009), *Abjectly Boundless: Boundaries, Bodies and Health Care* (Ashgate, 2010), and editor of *(Re)Thinking Violence in Health Care Settings: A Critical Approach* (Ashgate, 2011). He has presented at numerous national and international conferences. He has been appointed as Honorary Visiting Professor in Australia, the United States and the United Kingdom

Caroline Homer is Professor of Midwifery at the University of Technology Sydney, the Director of the Centre for Midwifery, Child and Family Health and the Director of Midwifery Studies in the Faculty of Nursing, Midwifery and Health at UTS. Caroline is currently leading research and consultancies into safety and quality in health care, models of maternity care including homebirth, Aboriginal maternal and infant health care, workforce issues for maternity care providers. She is also part of research teams developing a system to track severe maternal morbidity; and, testing new ways of providing maternity care. Caroline has been involved in the development of curricula and teaching midwifery students, both clinically and through UTS. She is an instructor in the Advanced Life Support in Obstetrics Course and the Maternity Emergency Course for the Council for Remote Area Nurses of Australia (CRANA). She is a member of the NSW Maternal and Perinatal Health Priority Taskforce which provides high level strategic advice to the NSW Minister for Health.

Andrew Long is Professor of Health Systems Research in the School of Healthcare, University of Leeds, UK. There he leads a research programme on health services evaluation and outcome measurement, centred on applied health research and research into practice.

Patrick O'Byrne is an Assistant Professor in the School of Nursing, Faculty of Health Sciences, at the University of Ottawa. His field of research and clinical practice is public health, particularly in relation to sexually transmitted infections and HIV. As part of this, he has been involved in various Canadian Institute of Health Research (CIHR) funded projects involving marginalized populations, such as, men who have sex with men (gay, bisexual, queer men), teens, swingers, and the homeless. Patrick has received a Governor General's Academic Gold Medal for this work and he is also the recipient of an Early Researcher Award from the Ministry of Research and Innovation (Government of Ontario).

Anne-Grete Sandaunet is a post-doctoral candidate at the Department of Sociology, Political Science and Community Planning, University of Tromsø, Norway. She has a main research interest in the sociology of illness. Her contributions to this area draw on explorations of breast cancer diagnosed women's use of online self-help groups and on the turn to Complementary and Alternative Medicine (CAM) among CFS/ME patients. Anne-Grete's research interests also include the sociology of professions. She is currently involved in research that explores the construction of professional roles in clinical contexts where decentralization of health care and multidisciplinary work represents important frames.

Stefan Timmermans is Professor of Sociology at UCLA Department of Sociology. His research draws from medical sociology and science studies and uses ethnographic and historical methods to address key issues in the for-profit US health care system. He has conducted research on medical technologies, health professions, death and dying, and population health. He is currently the medical sociology editor of the journal *Social Science & Medicine*.

Aksel Tjora is Professor of Sociology at the Norwegian University of Science and Technology (NTNU). His research focuses on the interaction between users and technologies in a number of areas, such as health, communication, architecture, music, as well as in organisations and public space, themes on which he has published widely internationally. Aksel has initiated a new thrust within sociology of health and illness in Norway, with an annual national health sociology conference and several edited books. He is also the editor of the *Norwegian Journal of Sociology*.

Philip Tovey is a health sociologist and Professor of Health and Wellbeing at the Faculty of Health and Social Care, the University of Hull, UK. He joined the faculty in 2010 from the University of Leeds. His first degree is in psychology and sociology and his PhD is in sociology. He has active research collaborations with universities in Brazil, India and Australia. He has been co-editor-in-chief of *Complementary Therapies in Medicine*. Philip's main research interest is the sociology of traditional, complementary and alternative medicine (TCAM). His work has been supported by around 20 external grants from a range of bodies including the ESRC, Medical Research Council (MRC), UK Department of Health and the British Academy. This has covered primary research in the UK, Australia, Pakistan, India and Brazil. The central element of this work is a critical engagement with processes of advocacy, utilisation and integration of TCAM globally. Much of the work has focused on these issues in relation to cancer. He has published widely; outputs include seven books.

Sarah Tyson is Professor of Rehabilitation in the School of Health, Sport and Rehabilitation Science, University of Salford, UK. Her research focuses upon stroke rehabilitation, and she uses a mixed methods approach to develop measurement tools and their application in practice. She has published widely in this field, and is President of the Society for Research in Rehabilitation.

Evan Willis is Professor of Sociology and Associate Dean (Regions) at La Trobe University. Over a long career, primarily as a medical sociologist, he has worked on a variety of topics including the division of labour in health care, occupational health and safety, complementary and alternative health care, RSI, evidence-based health care, genomics and the social relations of medical technology. His 1999 book, *Medical Dominance: The Division of Labour in Australian Health Care*, was, in 2003, voted by peers as one of the ten most influential books in Australian Sociology.

List of Abbreviations

ACOG	American College of Obstetricians and Gynaecologists
AMA	Australian Medical Association
BMA	British Medical Association
CAM	Complementary and Alternative Medicine
CPG	Clinical Practice Guidelines
EBHC	Evidence-based healthcare
EBM	Evidence-based medicine
EBNP	Evidence-based nursing practice
EBOT	Evidence-based occupational therapy
EBP	Evidence-based practice
EBPC	Evidence-based patient choice
HTA	Health Technology Assessment
NHS	National Health Service
RANZCOG	Royal Australian and New Zealand College of Obstetricians and Gynaecologists
RCT	Randomised controlled trial
WHO	World Health Organization

Chapter 1

A Critical Social Science
of Evidence-Based Healthcare

Alex Broom and Jon Adams

Introduction

In many respects evidence-based healthcare is neither new nor are its philosophical underpinnings unique. Getting the best knowledge to the right people in a timely fashion is commonsense. Yet, this basic principle reflects a broader social movement in knowledge production and dissemination that has been emerging for centuries. Scientific inquiry, as it were, has become more systematic, globally connected and protocol driven over the course of the twentieth century. While scientific discoveries in the nineteenth and early twentieth centuries still often occurred in the context of a sole or renegade researcher/practitioner, the latter part of the twentieth century witnessed the global streamlining, enhanced connectivity and dramatic institutionalisation of scientific knowledge production. This fundamentally changed the way both science and medicine were practiced in terms of research priorities and practice guidelines. While changes were occurring within the scientific community more broadly, 'modern' medicine, given its prominence in the community, became centre stage in this broader social movement and philosophical shift toward regulation, abstraction and systematisation in research and clinical practice. As the systematisation of healthcare developed and matured over the last few decades of the twentieth century we saw the institutional emergence of 'evidence-based medicine' (EBM), followed by 'evidence-based practice' (EBP), and then many other evidence-based models in the health and social care professions. This book is about these movements – which we put under the umbrella of 'evidence-based healthcare' (EBHC) – and setting a broad sociological platform from which to understand how these new knowledge technologies impact upon the practice of health care.

While there has been a significant shift in the definitions of, and rhetoric surrounding, the evidence-based social movements, the broad principles have remained relatively stable over time. In a well known maxim, EBM was articulated from an early stage of its development as 'the conscientious, explicit, and judicious use of current best evidence in making decisions about the care of individual patients' (Sackett et al. 1996, see also Evidence-Based Medicine

Working Group 1992). Now viewed as a sensible, perhaps uncontroversial, and certainly commonsense, statement, within the sociohistoric context that it was first articulated, it served as a timely warning that, despite the dramatic expansion of medical knowledge making in the twentieth century, methods of disseminating and utilising such knowledge internationally were limited if not non-existent for many areas of medicine. At the time, large numbers of clinicians did not follow the latest and most rigorous evidence, either due to lack of time, lack of expectation to be up-to-date, or lack of access to relevant evidence among other factors. Cochrane (1972) in particular highlighted the problem of a lack of up-to-date and high quality data for practicing clinicians, particularly in maternity care. Change was urgently needed and epidemiology began its rather dramatic ascendancy in the race to shape the form, representation and delivery of 'good medicine' in the twentieth and twenty-first centuries. Sackett's statement, as suggested, is quite simple, and understood within its socio-historic context, quite reasonable. Moreover, it conveys a seemingly benign concept. That is, until one considers the question of what constitutes 'evidence' and how the technologies of capture, synthesis and dissemination imbue and exclude certain ideas about the importance of certain types of knowledge (Holmes et al. 2006b).

Such historical calls for action from Cochrane, Guyatt and Sackett among others, have prompted action, evolved and even mutated into a wider complex system of global regulation of medical and health knowledge (Timmermans and Kolker 2004). Initial philosophical positions implicit in the 'first wave' EBM movement (Holmes et al. 2006a, Holmes et al. 2006b) were made explicit with the rapid formalisation and institutionalisation of the technologies and practices of knowledge synthesis (Borenstein and Hedges 2009, Higgins and Green 2011). That is, a sophisticated and powerful set of techniques around the production, assessment, and thus representation of medical knowledge – a process based largely on a hierarchy prioritising epidemiological/experimental designs (and often the synthesis of their outputs). Moreover, first wave EBM advocated the development of tools that are epistemologically consistent with the principles of epidemiology; tools that clinicians and clinicians-in-training could use to 'judge' the quality of evidence for themselves.

Central to the EBHC social movement has been the development and transcendence of meta-analysis (Borenstein and Hedges 2009, Moreira 2007) and different forms of critical evaluation of study design and trial quality including the Jadad and Pedro scales (see Bhogal et al. 2005, see also Jadad and Enkin 2007). It is worth noting that there was no meaningful debate around whether the development of a global system to collate and disseminate the rapidly expanding mass of health and medical knowledge was needed. It was needed, and urgently. Consider that between five and ten percent of all clinical trials published each year deal with cancer or cancer-related conditions, presenting oncology clinicians with well over 10,000 clinical trials annually (Ioannidis, Schmid and Lau 2000). Filtering even a small proportion of this information – not to mention assessing quality for use in everyday clinical work – is clearly implausible and unreasonable for oncology clinicians. The production of medical knowledge was (and in many respects still is) outdoing clinicians' capacity to use or make sense of it. Such conditions ensured the enthusiastic uptake amongst many stakeholders of an EBM-type strategy for knowledge filtering and treatment prioritisation. The fact that such 'filtering' and 'layering' was to be based on a very distinct and problematic epistemology (De Vries and Lemmens 2006, Goldenberg 2006, Gordon 2006, Holmes, Peron and O'Bryne 2006, Webb 2001) would present many stakeholders, including patients and clinicians, with a series of difficult questions in day-to-day care settings such as 'what is legitimate knowledge?', 'how important are population studies?' and 'how relevant is my or my patient's subjective experience?' (Broom and Tovey 2007b).

In many respects it is inevitable that the move to systematise expanding medical and health knowledge would lead to a crisis in 'what constitutes knowledge' (Mykhalovskiy and Weir 2004); a question far from clear in an increasingly pluralistic medical landscape (Broom and Tovey 2007a) particularly given the various patient movements supporting non-biomedical and non-evidence-based forms of care (Bakx 1991). Moreover, while there existed collective energy within the medical community focused on containing the growing corpus of research and controlling for quality, resistance and uncertainty persisted within medicine itself (Armstrong 2002, Pope 2003). Evidence-based – *from whose perspective?* – emerged as a key question that has persisted from the beginnings of the social movement to today (Greenhalgh 1999, Sullivan 2003). Evidence, according to what measures, also dominated discontents around EBHC. Yet, despite ongoing disputes within and outside medicine, the original EBM model quickly extended beyond the governance of practices within the medical profession and healthcare services.

Evidence-based paradigms now fundamentally shape the way health service providers, health funding bodies, governments and policy makers view 'effectiveness', and their willingness to fund and support interventions, practices, models of care and practitioner groups (Jackson and Scambler 2007, Webb 2001). EBHC and the various permutations thereof (EB practice, EB nursing practice, EB social work, EB decision making, EB physiotherapy, EB occupational therapy – the list goes on) are now shaping how we are treated, which treatments are funded, the character of illness experiences, quality of life, and ultimately, our survival chances. It is for this reason that it is vital that we explore and reveal the benefits and limitations of EBHC models in clinical context. Here we do not to dismiss the principles of the various forms of EBHC, denigrate key stakeholders, nor pursue an overly constructivist perspective common in the social sciences. Such a perspective would provide little room for acknowledgement of the legitimacy of objectivist or predictive techniques, and thus restrict constructive dialogue. Rather, we seek to examine how the principles, technologies and practices of 'evidence-based approaches' may allow certain things and promote certain understandings of health and illness while silencing others.

The Technologies of Knowledge and Consolidation of a Social Movement

As we shall see in the following chapters, the EBHC social movement has been successful largely due to the development of a sophisticated array of technologies and encoded practices that imbue particular values around the nature and production of knowledge (Broom, Adams and Tovey 2009, Timmermans and Berg 1997). That is, since the lexicon of EBM and EBP began to develop in the 1980s and 1990s we have seen the successful deployment and widespread uptake of formalised EBM technologies, design hierarchies and organisation structures that perpetuate their core principles and values. Meta-analysis, in particular, is one very effective facet of the multi-pronged program of 'knowledge contextualisation' promoted by key entities such as the Cochrane Collaboration, the Campbell Collaboration and the RAND Corporation. The construction of ideologically-infused technologies responsible for sorting the wheat from the chaff, so to speak, consolidated EBM-type models as central to judgements about the worthiness of studies and legitimacy of interventions (Moreira 2007). Various quality scales and systems of delineation emerged concurrently to the development of the aforementioned organisational entities to objectify and validate assessments. These scales – which have in turn been mimicked more recently for interpretive designs (The Joanna Briggs Institute 2011) – rate studies according to various features including randomisation, blinding, power and dropout among other things.

The trajectory towards evidence synthesis was swift in the 1990s with emphasis placed on consolidating an objective basis for synthesis, for example, effect sizes, within meta-analysis (Higgins and Green 2011, Jadad and Enkin 2007). This effectively created an enhanced a culture of polarisation in knowledge legitimacy – an evidence apartheid that many argue is politically driven and epistemologically reductive (Goldenberg 2006, Holmes et al. 2006a, Holmes et al. 2006b, Lambert 2006, Mykhalovskiy and Weir 2004). This positioned analytical/epidemiological design strategies as producing the most legitimate and accurate forms of medical knowledge (Broom, Barnes and Tovey 2004, Jackson and Scambler 2007). While the design priorities inherent in EBHC technologies do not explicitly marginalise interpretive designs, and thus qualitative insights and/or data, they do exclude interpretive designs from being part of the crux of a systematic review. By default, interpretive designs are reduced in their perceived significance for clinical work. In many established reviews of interventions interpretive data is not considered in the data meta-analysis. Descriptive/ interpretive design strategies may be present (often in background sections or as 'context') but do not inform the actual outcome. This has been a critical part of the epistemological dominance of analytical design strategies that still dominate medical research and the development of clinical guidelines.

There is no doubt that the original intention of the EBM entrepreneurs was to reduce the influence of bias, poor design and poorly run or analysed studies, so as to improve healthcare delivery (Cochrane 1972, Sackett et al. 1996). Moreover, the institutions that developed were aimed at improving cost-effectiveness by reducing the use of 'ineffective treatments'. In other words, these evidenced-based approaches were designed to protect patients and communities from being treated or receiving healthcare on the basis of poorly designed studies that may be harmful rather than beneficial. Of course, the problem that emerged was in what constituted 'poor design' and the philosophical conception of validity. Ultimately, a positivist epistemology dominated early EBM models and most EBHC models today, directing funding, governance and practice toward principles around population effects and distanced meta-analysis (Holmes et al. 2006a, Holmes et al. 2006b). Moves to systematise quality assessments and synthesise knowledge were represented as removing politics, poor techniques and human influence from the production and application of medical knowledge. Yet, such objectivities were illusory rather than reflected in the reality of knowledge work in medicine. Systems that rationalise quality and sort through the mass of healthcare information available are understandably appealing for many stakeholders, including managers and policy makers seeking to rationalise the delivery of certain interventions or services over others. As suggested, in the second half of the twentieth century, knowledge production (particularly publication in academic journals) was expanding dramatically and yet methods of information delivery, above and beyond individual clinicians reading studies and informing junior doctors, were lagging behind. The speed of knowledge production greatly outweighed the capacity of clinicians to understand, absorb and utilise knowledge. Moreover, most clinical programs did not, and still do not, provide rigorous training in study design and research methods. As such, a usable system of assessment, delivery and suitably institutionalised 'production houses', was met with significant enthusiasm from many quarters of the medical and healthcare establishment.

Professional Governance, Legitimacy and the Proliferation of EBHC

Politically and socially, the mid to late twentieth century was becoming increasingly risk adverse and market orientated, and there was increasing pressure for 'governance' in health service delivery and within the health and social care professions (Halligan and Donaldson 2001). Such agendas were complex and multifaceted, incorporating wider concerns over localised idiosyncrasies in health practice, cost blowouts, state-driven pressure for enhanced accountability, private sector drives for profit maximisation and a genuine concern for the widespread variations in care. Within 'other' health and social care professions – that is those other than medicine – considerable changes were taking place concurrent to the development and proliferation of EBM. Whilst medicine was the first professional and clinical body to explicitly push for rigorous across-the-board practice guidelines, hierarchies of evidence and a top-down model of managerial control over clinical practice, there have become a wide range of incentives from other health and social care professions to develop their own version of EBM. Being an 'evidence-based' profession has become critical for receiving funding, bolstering state legitimacy, achieving rhetorical legitimacy, gaining proximal credentialing and so on (Kessenich, Guyatt and DiCenso 1997, Richardson 2002, Webb 2001). Whether evidence-based nursing practice (Kessenich, Guyatt and DiCenso 1997) or evidence-based occupational therapy (Egan et al. 1998), health and social care professionals have come under pressure to replicate and transform EBM to fit their practices and shape processes of enhanced professionalisation and systematisation (Holmes, Perron and O'Byrne 2006). Moreover, such models have spread beyond state-supported and biomedically-credentialised practices to areas such as CAM, with the advent of evidence-based complementary medicine (Richardson 2002). Over the second half of the twentieth century nursing, physiotherapy, midwifery and occupational therapy have each gradually moved towards degree-based, regulated, nationally-credentialised and 'organised' professions with the development of practice guidelines in order to achieve professional credibility. An EBHC-type model has fed into each of these 'health professions' trajectories towards professionalisation and cultural legitimacy. Thus, the technologies developed initially for EBM have been drawn on, co-opted, and at times transformed, within the context of other professional groups. This has ultimately caused significant difficulties due to different ideological positions of the different health professions. Such developments are illustrative of the fact that advocates and proponents of 'first-wave' EBM have facilitated a flow-down effect which has shifted the rhetorical representation, and in many cases everyday practice, of many other health professional groups seeking enhanced credibility through 'consistency' in practice. Access to state resources has in turn become intimately intertwined with the espousal of a form of EBHC. As such, sociologically, EBHC models, including their devices and technologies, have come to dominate the regulation and centrality (or marginality) of different professional groups and thus accepted models of care and health care practices.

In many respects the success of the EBM movement and subsequent EBM-type models has been due to its ability to systematise, formalise and encode a complex value system that has now become the backbone of medical knowledge production (Timmermans and Berg 2003): the production of scales of assessment and hierarchies of evidence – or encoded knowledge. Organisationally and ideologically, proponents of EBHC have developed a coherent and systematised method of knowledge production and dissemination that seems from many positions to improve patient care, to reduce clinician uncertainty, and to provide enhanced evidence without the costs of additional studies (Andrews et al. 2006). Moreover, the principles of EBHC, could, it would seem, be applied to a wide range of health and social care professions. In a neo-liberal cultural shift, evident in many developed and some developing countries during the last two decades (Chomsky 1999), such guidelines provided an effective means of prioritising funding and offered a potential strategy for reducing litigation in increasingly privatised health services (Rosoff 2001). Thus, EBHC was highly attractive to many stakeholders including governments, policy makers, managers and private healthcare corporations. Yet, the discontent surrounding EBHC was evident in the experiences, reactions and perceptions of the two key players in healthcare delivery: patients and clinicians. Over the last few years there has been an emerging body of work, some from medicine and health and some from the social sciences, exploring a range of discontents regarding EBHC models at a grassroots level. Below, we provide a broad context to such debates.

Evidence-Based Healthcare and the Patient

Any model of knowledge production and dissemination, and clinical regulation has the greatest impact on those being treated and those doing the treating. We begin with the former. It goes without saying that pre-EBHC, many patients were given substandard, if not dangerous, forms of care due to an ineffective system of information delivery. The classic obstetrics case, pointed out by Archie Cochrane, that corticosteroids reduce the risk of babies dying from immaturity 30 to 50 per cent, illustrates the dangers of a lack of an institutionalised, systematic means of reviewing and dissemination evidence (Cochrane 1972). Because no systematic review of these trials had been published until 1989 – a process that would have identified a smaller well designed study showing powerful effect – most obstetricians had not realised that corticosteroids were so effective. As a result, thousands of babies had died unnecessarily. This is but one example of the flaws evident in historical practices of health knowledge production and utilisation that existed prior to the development of principles espoused by proponents of EBHC. In saying this, the current situation is quite distinct from that witnessed in the mid to late twentieth century. We now have a global system of evidence review, synthesis and dissemination and thus the new threat is that the principles of the original movement no longer resonate with patient experiences or perceptions of effectiveness (Broom and Tovey 2007b). Moreover, the reliance on cohort data, epidemiological design strategies and formalised information systems based on historical data, has the potential to remove the person (or aspects of personhood) from the healthcare process. This includes ideas about wellbeing, agency, belief, subjectivity and so on (Goldenberg 2006).

Patient-centred medicine (Bensing 2000) or evidence-based patient choice (Hope 1996) have in some respects been attempts to reconfigure the principles of the EBHC movements to centre more squarely on engaging patient perspectives once an 'evidence base' has been identified. To an extent such concepts have addressed some of the problems of the early application of EBM. Because of the push for trial data synthesis – rather than a focus on the meanings of illness and outcomes to different people and cultures – the focus in medicine moved even further away from the person to a focus on the condition or health issue. This mind-body split (the Cartesian dualism) already presented problems in the practice of medicine (Samson 1999). EBHC in many respects enhanced this issue through providing an even greater degree to abstraction – that is, from clinical practice and patient experience – through a focus on epidemiological and experiential designs.

Consumerism has become a powerful force in the mid to late twentieth century and the population-driven principles of EBM have, in some respects, operated counter to prevailing social forces espousing individualism, choice and a market economy (Slater 1997). That is, and particularly in western contexts, healthcare was increasingly viewed as a commodity to be purchased, placing pressure on health providers to adapt to the needs of consumers, rather than follow strictly the guidelines imposed by regulatory bodies or dominant professional organisations (Smith and Lipsky 1992). One example of this was the increasing provision of CAM in the private sector, despite a perceived lack of biomedical evidence for many CAMs, due to demand-based private provision of health services (Pelletier and Astin 2002). In this sense, the more market- and consumer-driven health systems of the US and Australia progressed more quickly than the more publicly orientated health systems of the UK and New Zealand in terms of treatment provisions based on the desires of patients in addition to those validated by 'evidence'. For example, private insurers began offering healing therapies in hospitals post surgery in the US regardless of the 'evidence base' available given the clear advantages in shorter stays in hospital. In this sense, market liberalisation reduced the capacity of the more extreme EBM stakeholders to dominate health rationing, at least in terms of healthcare delivery beyond the State.

This links to the reinsertion of the person in knowledge making and knowledge application in health and social care. Ultimately, private insurers and providers reacted to the strong demand for certain practices and ideas regardless of biomedical 'evidence base'. Simply put, it was not good business to withhold treatments that consumers wanted if such treatments were not overtly 'risky'. This included practices that enhanced everyday health and wellbeing (thus saving insurers money) that were considered by biomedical stakeholders amongst others as untestable in blinded, randomised clinical trials (aromatherapy massage is a good example in terms of private insurance rebates). Consumerism and private healthcare delivery allowed for the provision of practices, techniques and interventions that showed no or limited effect when 'measured' with biomedical study designs. Moreover, the availability of such products was restricted to the wealthy who could afford to purchase their own healthcare. In many respects those who paid the greatest price for the exclusion of non-evidence-based practices through EBHC type models in market capitalism were those at the bottom of the consumer ladder and those reliant on State resources. Thus forms of marginality, deprivation and exclusion interplay with the politics of EBHC, shaping patient experiences of and access to care.

This epistemological bias around knowledge legitimacy – the heavy reliance on abstracted, population-based trends – has and continues to sideline the *person*. Particularly important are the immeasurable features of health and wellbeing including such things as belief, spirituality, hope, intentionality, agency, community and personhood. These aspects may be controlled for (often as placebo) but more often than not remain unexamined as potent in their own right (Zahourek 2004). Moreover, within a cohort-focused model of evidence, aspects of human agency, subjectivity and self-determination lack meaningful recognition in the therapeutic process of the clinician-patient dynamic (Sullivan 2003). Such epistemological restrictions (the substitute of personhood for objective data) and ontological positions (my path/fate is identifiable by historical data) have been met with considerable resistance from many patients and people increasingly dissatisfied with biomedical interventions, particularly in the context of chronic illness. Communities are increasingly resisting exclusively biomedically-vetted interventions and are substituting and/or complementing them with self-care, preventative and complementary approaches to health and healing. As suggested above, such practices of self-care and resistance to EBHC models are largely in the realm of more affluent populations who can afford to resist dominant practices. While EBHC has provided a way of sorting and layering knowledge, its resonance with the experiences of those who are being treated has often been limited (Sullivan 2003). Questions around 'what works for me' or 'in my life' have been transformed into 'what works for my population of patients' and 'on average over their lives' (Broom and Tovey 2007b). While this has been the case for much longer than the existence of EBHC, this social movement has enhanced the imposition of depersonalisation and its discontents in healthcare delivery. This has impacted on the everyday work of health professionals, shaping their own ability to utilise subjective knowledge and intuition in practicing the art of healthcare.

Evidence-Based Healthcare and the Clinician

An extensive body of work has examined how clinicians view evidence, how EBHC is taught and implemented, and the question of what constitutes evidence in practice (Armstrong 2002, Broom, Adams and Tovey 2009, Broom and Adams 2010, Kessenich, Guyatt and DiCenso 1997, Pope 2003, Timmermans and Berg 1997). Our own research with staff specialists (consultants) and specialist nurses in Australia and in the United Kingdom has illustrated that while 'evidence', in the biomedical sense, is critical to everyday clinical work, EBHC models evade the actual subjectivities of clinical work and have in fact created new forms of clinical uncertainty (Broom, Adams and Tovey 2009, Broom and Tovey 2007a). Moreover, those in different hierarchical positions and professional groupings view the validity and importance of evidence in varied ways. In turn, as patients themselves seek to negotiate with clinicians regarding uncertainty over 'what constitutes evidence?' and 'what does it mean for me?', many clinicians are increasingly focusing on incorporating the 'human factor' into the decision-making and treatment process (Broom and Adams 2010). This points to the problematic of EBHC for clinicians working in many, if not all, sub-specialties of medicine.

Clinicians are faced with a plethora of ideological, epistemological and practical issues. The everyday realities of 'evidence' dissemination and the practice of medicine is that they *both* involve ongoing (but often implicit) value judgements about such things as the quality of evidence, risks, cost and patient preference (Gordon 2006, Moreira 2007). As Goldenberg suggests (2006), EBHC models often function to obscure such subjectivities and the social embeddedness of medical and healthcare knowledge.

For those working at the grassroots – rather than pushing professional or organisational objectives – there is consistent concern regarding the disconnection between EBHC (and processes of standardisation) and the actual character of contemporary medical work (Broom, Adams and Tovey 2009, De Vries and Lemmens 2006). This is particularly problematic given that the very value judgements and subjectivities that often go unrecognised in an EBHC framework are actually critically important skills in clinical practice with the constant emergence of new 'experimental' interventions and clinical data. What emerges, in a context of increased standardisation through EBHC, is a conflict between *res ipsa loquitur* ('the thing speaks for itself') and 'objective' scientific evidence. As Lambert (2006) emphasises, here lies the incommensurability between abstract epidemiological data and individual patient need and response. This has important implications not only for course of treatment, but what is defined as constituting a legitimate treatment in the first place (Lambert 2006).

The imposition of EBHC is partnered with diminished acceptance (or allowance of) the 'diagnostic art' or clinical judgement (Lambert 2006). Enhanced therapeutic rationality through standardisation, as encouraged within EBM models, may thus silence the individual clinician and the patient, by simultaneously suppressing the role of illness narratives and the 'expert eye' in medical work (Greenhalgh 1999). As Goldenberg (2006) suggests, an EBM framework tends to ignore the phenomenology of illness; the embodied, experiential facets of 'being treated' (the patient's experience) and 'treating' (the doctor's experience). Giving these philosophical, regulatory and practical concerns, it is perhaps unsurprising that EBHC is not always well received and can be difficult to actualise in clinical contexts (De Vries and Lemmens 2005, Lambert 2006). For example, exactly how differently positioned clinicians manage the practice of EBM; how they utilise forms of expertise in clinical practice; and, how they augment this with clinical intuition is largely unknown.

More recently, there has been a growing interest in the tensions between therapeutic rationality and clinical autonomy (Armstrong 2002). At one level, EBM has provided a specialty-specific method of professional control within medicine whereby research or medical elites strongly influence practitioners through clinical practice guidelines, treatment protocols and organisational information systems. Indeed, it has been argued that EBM represents a strategy for defending collective autonomy through restricting the individual freedoms of practitioners (Armstrong 2002).

The degree to which such trajectories toward therapeutic rationality and regulatory systematisation have been achieved (and the responses of different practitioner groups) has been well-examined by medical sociologists. For example, in his study of primary care physicians' management of depression and the impact of EBM therein, Armstrong (2002) illustrated a disconnect between formalised

EBM approaches and individual clinical decisions. Whilst EBM, Armstrong posits, is largely dependent on stimulating a critical 'moment of change' whereby one behaviour gives way to the other (that is, new evidence results in use of a different treatment), continuity, stability and subjectivities persist in primary care contexts. Armstrong (2002) argues that the persistence of individual judgement and situated decision-making is rationalised by doctors through the deployment of notions of uniqueness, indeterminacy, and the need for patient centredness. As such, we see the emergence of a counter-balance to EBM (also feeding into contemporary consumerist sentiment), to protect the integrity of individual clinical judgement. Armstrong (2002) characterises EBM and 'patient centredness' as playing concurrent, albeit potentially conflicting, roles in achieving and securing clinical power and autonomy in primary care.

In another key study, Pope (2003) utilises a social movements framework to examine EBM as perceived by urological and gynaecological/pelvic surgeons. In her analysis, Pope identifies the highly instinctual and contingent nature of these surgical sub-specialties, highlighting key sites of resistance to formalised training and established procedure. It was discovered that formalised accounts or evidence were regularly dismissed, and surgeons followed a model of 'experientially-learned practice', focusing on the 'how' (the doing of surgery), rather than the 'what' (the most effective procedure to use) (Pope, 2003).

Both these studies highlight strategies of coping with (and resisting) the increasing regulation and systematisation in medicine including the strategic re-emphasis on the importance of tacit, experiential knowledge as critical to medical work (see also Greenhalgh et al. 2008). These two studies illustrate the deployment of rhetorical and practical strategies to counter the threat of EBM including expositions of surgery as art or experiential and general practice as individualised and patient centred. Such practices are examples of intra-specialty defence against increased therapeutic rationality as promoted by EBM and its various manifestations. However, it should also be emphasised that effects may vary among differently positioned clinicians in the imposition of an EBM model. Highlighted by Friedson (2001) in his work on professions, rather than having linear effects (power reduction/consolidation), regulatory frameworks like EBM may actually create internal status differences within medicine resulting in a reduction of clinical autonomy (or proletarianisation) for some and increased status (including career advancement) for others. Specifically, binary notions of power reduction/proletarianisation through bureaucratic rationality may not hold up in grassroots clinical contexts where clinicians are strategically adapting to organisational and ideological shifts.

However, whilst practicing physicians may engage in forms of resistance in order to retain the perceived integrity of their medical work, the implications of EBHC for the training of doctors and the shaping of expertise remains a critical issue for the medical community, though there has been little sociological work in the area. Drawing on a study of paediatric residents in the US, Timmermans and Angell (2001) found that EBM may actually increase uncertainty in junior doctors due to an increased reliance on information systems and epidemiology. Furthermore, and extending on the point made above, EBM acted to solidify the hierarchical relationships between consultants and junior doctors, reducing questioning, critical thinking and the process of learning through experience (Timmermans and Angell 2001). What these studies tell us is that EBHC is having unintended consequences. These include potentially increasingly uncertainty, reducing autonomy and limiting a sense of agency within healthcare 'transactions'. While the benefits of systematisation are quite clear, the limitations are often left out of the equation, so to speak. Ultimately, and as shown in each of the following chapters, we argue that EBHC should be critically examined in terms of how it impacts on the day-to-day lives of patients and clinicians. Social science offers the unique methodological tools and the conceptual basis to provide such insight.

A Critical Social Science of Evidence-Based Healthcare?

Establishing a critical sociology of EBHC that speaks to a range of audiences is necessary for a number of reasons. First there has been relatively limited exposure within the health and social care professions to a critical social science approach to evidence and the production of knowledge. Critique has tended to come from those working within philosophy which has been traditionally less focused on exploring clinically-embedded case studies of the complexity of knowledge. EBHC is now a global web of institutions, gurus, technologies, devices, policies and is defining the healthcare we receive (or do not receive, as the case may be) when we seek help. As a social movement, evidence-based models are defining what it is to be a patient and what it is like to be a clinician. It has, and continues to, produce, enhance and perpetuate some of the classic power struggles in the health and wellbeing professions and in the academic community. Nursing-medicine, physiotherapy-chiropractic, complementary medicine-medicine – these relationships are each to some degree being shaped by claims about, and perspectives on, evidence. And, particular kinds of evidence. Age-old tensions between midwife and physician, between complementary practitioner and doctor, are being played out through the politics of study designs, epistemological supremacy and the 'science wars'-type battle between interpretivism and objectivitism. Such classic debates between quantitative measurement and the interpretation of subjective experience do little to assist those at the grassroots trying to get better or help people get better. This juggernaut that has entered global discourse is feeding tensions between those in support of ideas about subjective wellbeing rather that quality adjusted life years and those in support of human agency and self-determination rather than epidemiological predictors of survival. It is thus time to move towards a critical sociology of EBHC that can provide a sense of the social embeddedness of knowledge; that is, one that rests in a political and cultural basis of diverse claims to legitimacy. This is not a relativist positioning but a way of reinserting what already exists in health and social care – the human elements whether patient, practitioner or carer related.

This text is not a criticism of EBHC. Each author – some actively working and researching in clinical contexts, with social science backgrounds, and others operating in academic contexts – value and acknowledge the production and use of multiple forms of knowledge. Rather, this book and each author seek to outline a way of understanding evidence in a particular context. Together, these works assert the need to understand the potencies and limitations of particular forms of knowledge as well as voice clinical and personal discontents with a linear application of knowledge. Ultimately, some form of knowledge production and dissemination is critical and thus our purpose is not to dismantle but instead to contextualise, balance and emphasise some often marginalised voices in the debate about EBHC.

Outline of the Chapters

In Part I of this collection entitled 'Evidence in Cultural and Theoretical Context' we present two broad perspectives on the impacts of EBHC for medicine and the health sciences. Chapter 2, co-written by one of the founding sociologists of EBM, Stefan Timmermans, explores uncertainty within the context of the EBM movement and the degree to which forms of systematisation and standardisation actually feed into, shape and problematise medical training. Drawing on interviews with paediatric residents (in newborn units, endocrinology, haematology–oncology, paediatric intensive care, paediatric surgery and an emergency department), the focus here is on the practical problematic of an individual's ability to absorb EBM into the practice of medicine. Timmermans shows that, contrary to EBM's quest for certainty, EBM-in-practice unintentionally generates new forms of uncertainty. Moreover, however, Timmermans is careful to point out that the pursuit of disembedded, 'de-humanised', forms of knowledge production does not necessarily lead to detached or de-humanised approaches to healthcare delivery among practitioners.

Chapter 3, authored by Dave Holmes and Patrick O'Byrne, provides an engaging critique of EBHC as a political movement that ultimately seeks to dominate (reductively) the production of knowledge. That is, a form of governmentality that does not 'stop people speaking' but asks that they 'speak in particular ways'. They argue that evidence-based medicine has been about epistemological dominance and is flawed in its politicised dependence on epidemiological study designs. The authors provide a sophisticated and engaging call for resistance and a reconfiguration of EBHC. The authors advocate for a form of EBHC that accommodates plural, multi-layered and epistemologically diverse sources of knowledge about the world. Within this chapter, EBM in particular is conceptualised as an imperialistic form of stratification that produces a polarised culture of evidence legitimacy. The authors utilise Deleuze and Guattari's concept of the war machine as a means of countering EBMs dominance in knowledge making.

In Part II, 'Evidence in the Clinic', we move to an examination of EBHC in the context of three specific (and quite different) clinical contexts. These include abdominal aortic aneurysm, neuro-rehabilitation and medical oncology/ haematology respectively in Norway, Britain and Australia. These three cross-cultural settings provide a series of critical examinations of how 'evidence', in the clinic, becomes transformed and reconfigured by different actors and stakeholders – that is, the specificities of what evidence does and becomes when it reaches clinical contexts.

Berit Brattheim, Arild Faxvaag and Aksel Tjora, in Chapter 4, examine, in the context of the surgical treatment of abdominal aortic aneurysm in Norway, how evidence for endovascular repair (EVAR) develops within a particular social, material, technological, and organisational context. The authors highlight the extent to which knowledge is produced within a communal context and thus how the sociality of clinical practice creates evidence. Beyond mere adopters of evidence-based practice, the authors argue that, within the communal context, clinicians are equally knowledge (and evidence) producers.

In Chapter 5, Flynn and colleagues engage in an examination of the dialectic between explicit/encoded knowledge (promoted by EBHC trajectories) and tacit/ embedded forms of knowledge in the UK. Taking neurorehabilitation as their case in point, they explore the ways in which 'concrete' measures are subjected to interpretation, individual perspective and contextual circumstances. This chapter illustrates how encoding at a theoretical level (or at a policy level) results in the re-contextualisation in clinical practices and thus how evidence-based guidelines will, necessarily, always constitute a partial rendering of the complete knowledge of clinicians. That is, while standardisation provides an explicit sense of coherence, the ways in which the tools of standardisation are utilised, co-opted and transfigured in different clinical contexts illustrates the inevitability of tacit knowledge and intuitive practice. Such findings remind us of the problematic of attempting to impose a rational system that irrationally excludes human subjectivities and their capacity to utilise intuitive knowledge effectively.

In Chapter 6, we contribute a chapter which focuses on how evidence is viewed, presented and utilised differentially in medical oncology and haematology. We follow the respective rationales of specialists and nurses for what constitutes 'good enough' evidence, illustrating differentiation in perspective, and how the histories of these specialties, institutional hierarchies, and inter-professional dynamics shape their accounts. That is, their perspectives on what constitutes 'enough evidence' to warrant using an intervention on a cancer patient. Our findings illustrate that, in practice, what is presented, talked about, and utilised as evidence, is highly differentiated between specialities, between individual clinicians and according to hierarchy. We draw on and extend the concept of 'localised universality' (see Timmermans and Berg 1997) – the imposition of idiosyncratic standards and protocols within an individual institution – to illustrate the importance of culture within particular medical specialties and institutional hierarchies as shaping what constitutes 'good evidence'.

Part III is titled 'Evidence on the Margins' and focuses on a critical social science of specific sites of epistemological and actual marginality, in terms of state support and in the context of contested legitimacy. Specifically, this section examines ideas about evidence from the perspectives of complementary and alternative practitioners, midwives, and patients, each of whom remain in peripheral positions in terms of their contribution to, perspectives on, and role in the production of evidence.

Chapter 7, by Kevin Dew, examines the interplay between uncertainty and standardisation, taking a group of New Zealand General Practitioners' engagement with CAM as a case study. Dew shows how the inevitable uncertainty in GPs everyday work – and the inability of the biomedical model and EBM to capture such uncertainties – may create a point of identity crisis that leads them to engage in CAM models of care. This rupture is transformative, and Dew argues enables a (professional) biographical development of sorts, reflecting the persistent discontent (see also Armstrong 2002) among many GPs with the trajectory of EBM. The search for an approach to care that accommodates multiple forms of knowledge, incorporates patient subjectivities, and accommodates 'uncertainty' underpins the GPs accounts examined in this chapter.

In Chapter 8, Alex Broom and Philip Tovey explore how patients engage with and perceive notions of 'evidence' and 'effectiveness'. Drawing on the controversial issue of complementary medicines in cancer care, this chapter explores how patients themselves balance what they 'know in themselves' *vis-à-vis* 'what is known their bodies will do' (in terms of biomedical evidence). This chapter illustrates the limits of probabilities and statistical predictions in the context of a strong patient focus on hope, agency and self-determination. While it is shown that terminality shapes patient engagement with biomedical evidence, it is also shown that here remains a strong push for reinserting the individual into the 'evidence equation'. This desire, on the part of cancer patients, is embedded in dialectical tension between individuation and depersonalisation. That is, the desire for an approach to care that is not exclusively about biomedical 'effectiveness' *or* the life world of the individual cancer patient. Rather, the study of these patients highlights how intuitive and embodied knowledges should be intertwined with, and presented alongside abstracted, population-based biomedical evidence.

In Chapter 9, by Caroline Homer and Alex Broom, the focus is on the relationship of midwifery to the politics of evidence and therapeutic legitimacy. This chapter examines the homebirth debate in Australia, sketching the historical and contemporary sociopolitical factors that shape the production, use, co-option, or refutation of evidence. This chapter traces the historical struggles between obstetrics and midwifery and shows how the parallel evolution of these disciplines frame current tensions around evidence and risk in the context of maternity care.

The final chapter, written by Evan Willis and Anne-Grete Sandaunet, provides a summary and overview of some potential future research directions for the study of EBHC as well as highlighting the political character of health delivery. Specifically, they draw on three case studies – breast cancer screening, prostate cancer screening and CAM integration – to outline a series of questions in need of further exploration. The cross-national differences in utilisation of screening for breast and prostate cancer are revealing in terms of the shaping of health service delivery according to belief, risk, litigation and political power, rather than actual evidence of effectiveness. Ultimately, these cases are used to illustrate the challenges facing EBHC in relation to issues of power and political influence – challenges that are likely to get more and more significant in a twenty-first century given a broader waning in support for a purely biomedical conception of knowledge production and therapeutic effectiveness.

Acknowledgements

Thanks to Carla Meurk for her fantastic help with putting together this collection.

References

Adams, J. 2001. General practitioners, evidence-based medicine and complementary therapies. *Complementary Therapies in Medicine*, 8(4), 248–52.

Andrews, G., Simonella, L., Lapsley, H., Sanderson K. and March, L. 2006. Evidence-based medicine is affordable: The cost-effectiveness of current compared with optimal treatment in rheumatoid and osteoarthritis. *The Journal of Rheumatology*, 33(4), 671–80.

Armstrong, D. 2002. Clinical autonomy, individual and collective. *Social Science and Medicine*, 55(10), 1771–7.

Bakx, K. 1991. The 'eclipse' of folk medicine in western society. *Sociology of Health and Illness*, 13(1), 20–38.

Barry, A. 2006. The role of evidence in alternative medicine. *Social Science and Medicine*, 62(11), 2646–57.

Bensing, J. 2000. Bridging the gap: The separate worlds of evidence-based medicine and patient-centered medicine. *Patient Education and Counselling*, 39(1), 17–25.

Bhogal, S., Teasell, R., Foley, N. and Speechley, M. 2005. The PEDro scale provides a more comprehensive measure of methodological quality than the Jadad Scale in stroke rehabilitation literature. *Journal of Clinical Epidimiology*, 58(7), 668–73.

Borenstein, M. and Hedges, L. 2009. *Introduction to Meta-Analysis*. Chichester: John Wiley and Sons.

Broom, A. and Adams, J. 2010. The reconfiguration of expertise in oncology: The practice of prediction and articulation of indeterminacy in medical consultations. *Qualitative Health Research*, 20(10), 1433–45.

Broom, A., Adams, J. and Tovey, P. 2009. Evidence-based healthcare in practice: A study of clinical resistance, professional deskilling, and inter-specialty differentiation in oncology. *Social Science and Medicine*, 68(1), 192–200.

Broom, A., Barnes, J. and Tovey, P. 2004. Introduction to research methods in complementary medicine. *Complementary Therapies in Medicine*, 12(2), 165–73.

Broom, A. and Tovey, P. 2007a. Therapeutic pluralism? Evidence, power and legitimacy in UK cancer services. *Sociology of Health and Illness*, 29(3), 551–69.

Broom, A. and Tovey, P. 2007b. The dialectical tension between individuation and depersonalisation in cancer patients' mediation of complementary, alternative and biomedical cancer treatments. *Sociology*, 41(6), 1021–39.

Cochrane, A. 1972. *Effectiveness and Efficiency.* London: Nuffield Provincial Hospitals Trust.

Chomsky, N. 1999. *Profit Over People: Neoliberalism and Global Order*. London: Seven Stories Press.

De Vries, R. and Lemmens, T. 2006. The social and cultural shaping and medical evidence. *Social Science and Medicine*, 62(11), 2694–706.

Egan, M., Dubouloz, C., von Zweck, C. and Vallerand, J. 1998. The client-centred evidence-based practice of occupational therapy. *Canadian Journal of Occupational Therapy*, 65(3), 136–43.

Evidence-Based Medicine Working Group. 1992. Evidence-based medicine: A new approach to teaching the practice of medicine. *Journal of the American Medical Association*, 268(17), 2420–25.

Freidson, E. 2001. *Professionalism: The Third Logic.* Chicago: University of Chicago.

Goldenberg, M. 2006. On evidence and evidence-based medicine: Lessons from the philosophy of science. *Social Science and Medicine*, 62(11), 2621–32.

Gordon, E. 2006. The political contexts of evidence-based medicine: Policymaking for daily hemodialysis. *Social Science and Medicine*, 62(11), 2707–19.

Greenhalgh, T. 1999. Narrative based medicine in an evidence based world. *British Medical Journal*, 318(7179), 323–5.

Greenhalgh, J., Flynn, R., Long, A. and Tyson S. 2008. Tacit and encoded knowledge in the use of standardised outcome measures in multidisciplinary team decision making: A case study of in-patient neurorehabilitation. *Social Science and Medicine*, 67(1), 183–94.

Halligan, A. and Donaldson, L. 2001. Implementing clinical governance: Turning vision into reality. *British Medical Journal*, 322, 1413.

Higgins, J. and Green, S. (eds) 2011. *Cochrane Handbook for Systematic Reviews of Interventions Version 5.1.0.* [Online]. Available at: www.cochrane-handbook.org [accessed: 20 September 2011].

Holmes, D., Perron, R. and O'Byrne, P. 2006. Evidence, virulence, and the disappearance of nursing knowledge: A critique of the evidence-based dogma. *Worldviews on Evidence-Based Nursing*, 3(3), 95–102.

Holmes, D., Murray, S., Perron, A. and Rail, G. 2006a. Towards an understanding of the politics of 'evidence'. *International Journal of Evidence-Based Health Care*, 4(4), 394–5.

Holmes, D., Murray, S., Perron, A. and Rail, G. 2006b. Deconstructing the evidence-based discourse in health sciences: Truth, power, and fascism. *International Journal of Evidence-Based Health Care*, 4(3), 180–86.

Hope, T. 1996. *Evidence-based Patient Choice*. London: King's Fund.

Ioannidis, J., Schmid, C. and Lau, J. 2000. Meta-analysis in hematology and oncology. *Hematology/Oncology Clinics of North America*, 14(4), 973–91.

Jackson, S. and Scambler, G. 2007. Perceptions of evidence-based medicine: Traditional acupuncturists in the UK and resistance to biomedical modes of evaluation. *Sociology of Health and Illness*, 29(3), 412–29.

Jadad, A. and Enkin, M. 2007. *Randomized Controlled Trials: Questions, Answers and Musings*. 2nd edition. Oxford: Blackwell.

Kessenich, C., Guyatt, G. and DiCenso, A. 1997. Teaching nursing students evidence-based nursing. *Nurse Educator*, 22(6), 25–9.

Lambert, H. 2006. Accounting for EBM: Notions of evidence in medicine. *Social Science and Medicine*, 62(11), 2633–45.

Moreira, T. 2007. Entangled evidence: Knowledge making in systematic reviews in healthcare. *Sociology of Health and Illness*, 29(2), 180–97.

Mykhalovskiy, E. and Weir, L. 2004. The problem of evidence-based medicine. *Social Science and Medicine*, 59(5), 1059–69.

Pelletier, K. and Astin, J. 2002. Integration and reimbursement of complementary and alternative medicine by managed care and insurance providers: 2000 update and cohort analysis. *Alternative Therapies in Health and Medicine*, 8(1), 38–9.

Pope, C. 2003. Resisting evidence: The study of evidence-based medicine as a contemporary social movement. *Health*, 7(3), 267–82.

Richardson, J. 2002. Evidence-based complementary medicine: Rigor, relevance, and the swampy lowlands. *The Journal of Alternative and Complementary Medicine*, 8(3), 221–3.

Rosoff, A. 2001. Evidence-based medicine and the law: The courts confront clinical practice guidelines. *Journal of Health Politics, Policy and Law*, 26(2), 327–68.

Sackett, D., Rosenberg, W., Gray, M., Haynes, B. and Richardson, S. 1996. Evidence-based medicine: What it is and what it isn't. *British Medical Journal*, 312(7050), 71–2.

Samson, C. 1999. Biomedicine and the body, in *Health Studies: A Critical and Cross-Cultural Reader*, edited by C. Samson. Oxford: Blackwell.

Slater, D. 1997. *Consumer Culture and Modernity*. Cambridge: Polity Press.

Smith, S. and Lipsky, M. 1992. Privatization in health and human services: A critique. *Journal of Health Politics, Policy and Law*, 17(2), 233–54.

Sullivan, M. 2003. The new subjective medicine: Taking the patient's point of view on health care and health. *Social Science and Medicine*, 56(7), 1595–604.

The Joanna Briggs Institute. 2011. *Appraise Evidence*. [Online]. Available at: http://www.joannabriggs.edu.au/Appraise%20Evidence [accessed: 20 September 2011].

Timmermans, S. and Angell, A. 2001. Evidence-based medicine, clinical uncertainty, and learning to doctor. *Journal of Health and Social Behaviour*, 42(4), 342–59.

Timmermans, S. and Berg, M. 1997. Standardization in action: Achieving local universality through medical protocols. *Social Studies of Science*, 27(2), 273–305.

Timmermans, S. and Berg, M. 2003. *The Gold Standard: The Challenge of Evidence-Based Medicine and Standardization in Health Care*. Philadelphia: Temple.

Timmermans, S. and Kolker, E. 2004. Evidence-based medicine and the reconfiguration of medical knowledge. *Journal of Health and Social Behavior*, 45, 177–93.

Tovey, P. and Broom, A. 2007. Oncologists' and specialist cancer nurses' approaches to complementary and alternative medicine use and their impact on patient action. *Social Science and Medicine*, 64(12), 2550–64.

Villanueva-Russell, Y. 2005. Evidence-based medicine and its implications for the profession of chiropractic. *Social Science and Medicine*, 60(3), 545–61.

Webb, S. 2001. Some considerations on the validity of evidence-based practice in social work. *British Journal of Social Work*, 31(1), 57–79.

Zahourek R. 2004. Intentionality forms the matrix of healing: A theory. *Alternative Therapies in Health and Medicine*, 10(6), 40–49.

PART I
Evidence in Cultural
and Theoretical Context

Chapter 2

Evidence-Based Medicine, Clinical Uncertainty, and Learning to Doctor

Stefan Timmermans and Alison Angell

Introduction

Since the early 1990s, the health care field has embarked on a standardisation movement under the banner of evidence-based medicine (EBM). According to the proponents of EBM, every decision a doctor makes on behalf of a patient should be supported with scientific evidence. The reliance on scientific evidence in medicine goes back at least two centuries to the Parisian schools of medicine (Foucault 1973) and standardisation has been used repeatedly in the past to consolidate the power of the medical profession (Starr 1982).

Yet, the scale and scope of standardising medical practice on scientific grounds is new. EBM relies largely on clinical practice guidelines and research protocols to disseminate proven (that is, supported with randomised clinical trials) diagnostic and therapeutic knowledge. Such guidelines offer step-by-step instructions on the most intimate details of medical care.

Because EBM centres on information gathering and evaluation, several medical educators have suggested an evidence-based curriculum and training to teach students medicine (see, for example, Ghali et al. 2000). Such curricula rest on a simple principle: instead of relying on how experienced clinicians order them to treat patients, 'students of health professions should be encouraged to ask every day, "What's the evidence?"' (Eisenberg 1999: 1868). Educators define EBM as a paradigm shift with three tenets: the integration of research based information in clinical practice, the realisation that pathophysiology is insufficient for the practice of clinical medicine, and the acquisition of methodological and statistical skills to evaluate studies. These three premises contrast with past training practices where medical knowledge transfer depended on the teacher's individual clinical experience and authority, where pathophysiology provided the foundation for clinical practice, and gaps in knowledge were filled with an experience generated common sense (Friedland 1999).

Frederic Hafferty notes that the rise of EBM might have repercussions for the study of medical school socialisation:

> We might want to revisit the writings of Renée Fox, Donald Light, and others on
> the nature and impact of uncertainty in medical work and question whether the

> deployment of research protocols and the use of report cards is generating a new
> definition of uncertainty in medical practice. (Hafferty 2000: 252)

Indeed, from a sociological perspective the widespread dissemination of EBM in medical education could be regarded as a means to alleviate the uncertainty inherent in medical knowledge (Good 1998). In her landmark article on training for uncertainty, Fox argued that students were overwhelmed by the vast amounts of knowledge to master and the many unknowns in the medical knowledge base (Fox 1957). Clinical practice guidelines and other standardised research-based learning tools not only summarise the literature in an easily accessible format but also guide the budding physician through the clinical encounter. Standardised instruments could then be the definitive answer to the problem of clinical uncertainty. Yet, the scant preliminary evidence shows that the link between EBM and residency training is not obvious (Bazarian et al. 1999). Although medical students might benefit from an EBM based medical curriculum, the immediate demands of residents on the ward seem to make critically appraising the literature before decision making unrealistic.

What, then, does this flow of EBM mean for medical socialisation and the acquisition of medical knowledge? We investigated how residents understand EBM and whether it applies to their own daily practice of managing the uncertainty of medicine. The chapter consists of three parts: first, we explain residents' understanding and practice of EBM, second, we discuss how EBM relates to clinical uncertainty, and finally, we investigate the relationship between research-based and experience-based knowledge.

Fieldwork

We interviewed 17 paediatric residents from two medical programmes about their experiences with EBM. Brandeis University's institutional review board approved this project. Both programmes were part of large, urban hospitals affiliated with academic institutions. As residents, our respondents had finished four years of medical school and were at different stages of three years of rotations in different clinical paediatric specialties. Most of the respondents were in their mid-twenties and white (three Asian respondents). The gender distribution was nine male and eight female residents. Eight respondents were in their first year of residency, two in the second year, five in the third year, and two chief residents were in their fourth year. Their rotations at the time of the interview varied from the newborn unit, endocrinology, haematology–oncology, paediatric intensive care, paediatric surgery, to the emergency department.

Potential respondents received a notice about the study from the chief resident. They then contacted the researchers and set-up an interview time. Even with the blessing of the attending, it remained difficult and time-consuming to access the residency programmes. Chief residents remained protective of the residents' time.

We managed to interview 45 per cent of the residents in both programmes. No one refused the interview after contacting us. The interviews were audio-recorded and lasted approximately one hour, with a few interviews lasting up to two and a half hours. All respondents were asked similar questions aimed at generating detailed stories but not necessarily in the same wording and sequence. The interviews were transcribed and went through successive rounds of open, selective, and axial coding (Strauss 1987). Residents' excerpts presented here have been anonymised through the use of a pseudonym.

Practicing Evidence-Based Medicine

The role of evidence-based medicine during resident training is defined by where a resident seeks information and how confident he or she feels to act on that information. In most rotations the residents have some autonomy about patient care: they are required to diagnose and work-up patients, monitor their hospital stay and order laboratory tests and medications. Since a resident has a MD degree and wears the clothes and paraphernalia of a hospital physician, patients expect medical competence. In this section we ask: how does EBM feature in the socialisation of doctoring?

All residents we interviewed stated that, in Dr Weiss' words, 'the new age of medicine is going toward EBM'. The two training programmes reflected that trend. They had an active lecture series, and had recently retooled their traditional journal clubs to make EBM more central. Chief residents, supervising attendings, and even pharmaceutical representatives recommended EBM. In one of the programmes, for example, an attending proposed having a librarian–researcher armed with an on-line computer present at morning meetings to provide EBM on the spot. As we will explore in more detail below, EBM was integrated in a hierarchical supervisory relationship: attendings would routinely request evidence before decision-making. Pharmaceutical reps would try to convince residents to use their drug for new applications while showing them research evidence published in major medical journals.

Steeped in an EBM environment, all residents reported that, at least occasionally, they 'did' EBM. They agreed that practicing EBM implied coming up with the best answer to a clinical diagnostic or treatment question. The best solution entailed patient management that was backed up with recently published research by authorities in the field. EBM offers the resident a written rationale for patient decisions and this justification is viewed as an alternative to choosing treatments based on anecdotal evidence and personal experience. Importantly, the respondents sharply bifurcated based on what kinds of literature they considered evidence and what should be done with it. We identified two key orientations to EBM: 11 residents relied on the evidence as librarians and six others utilised the literature more as researchers.

Librarian residents expanded the source material that qualifies for EBM. For the majority of residents, doing EBM meant consulting any published resource, including using computerised research databases. The information became authoritative from its text format, the institutional affiliation of its author and the journal. When asked for an instance of EBM, Dr Di Maio gave an example of checking the literature for a young patient who had been bitten by a parrot. He wondered whether parrot bites warrant special antibiotic treatment. A review article explained that, in contrast to dog bites, no antibiotic treatment is required for avian bites, but that the doctor should check for some typical infections. Although the article provided Dr Di Maio with guidance on a topic he did not know much about, it was not based on a systematic review of epidemiological literature.

In line with their broad criteria for EBM, librarian residents relied largely on 'cheat books', textbooks, guidelines and review articles. Several residents pulled a dog-eared copy of *The Harriet Lane Handbook: A Manual for Pediatric House Officers* (Siberry and Iannone 2000) out of their pocket. One resident lauded the book as 'the bible for paediatric residents'. Harriet Lane was mainly used to check medication dosages for children but it also contained a number of elementary protocols on how to treat common ailments. The next lines of defence for librarians were the thick, general textbooks that are strewn over the different paediatric wards. The 600 plus pages of the *Manual of Pediatric Therapeutics* (Graef 1997), for example, provides a basic orientation on how to handle most common disorders with some general explanation, but it is less up-to-date and comprehensive than some of the other sources. The most sophisticated literature sources consulted by librarians consisted of on-line protocols provided by professional organisations such as the American Academy of Paediatrics. On a similar level were review articles published in leading paediatric journals that critically assessed the state of the field and the strength of the evidence. When reading such articles, librarians skimmed the methodology and focused on the conclusion and findings.

Librarians consulted review articles, textbooks and guidelines because they provided quick answers to clinical questions. Most admitted that evaluating a primary study took too much time. Library residents frequently asked an attending for advice before approaching the literature as a principle time saving strategy. Dr Cole explained: 'Unfortunately, the way it works on the floor most of the time, because we are so busy, we can't fully research a topic. A more efficient way is to reach for help'. Library residents reserved literature searches for rare cases and for presentations in front of superiors. They stressed that time in the library was time spent away from the patient. Librarians found much evidence via the database MD Consult. This user-friendly database offered the advantage of providing full-text, on-line accessibility and was also linked to some major textbooks.

The core of EBM for librarian residents was the pragmatic reliance on literature to quickly solve the dilemma at hand. For that reason, librarians thought that medicine had always been steeped in EBM. Dr Cole noted:

I think it is like a new term for what medicine is and always has been: using the literature to come up with the best intervention. It is just that things have gotten sloppy, in that people are just going off their own experience and not using the literature to look critically. I feel like this new movement is a reinstitution of this whole idea.

In contrast to the residents who used the literature as a librarian, a minority of residents took the core of EBM to mean that the physician acted more as a researcher who actively evaluates and interprets the literature. Residents who professed to be more familiar with EBM specified that merely checking published literature is insufficient; EBM implies a critical assessment of available evidence in a meta-analysis. Ideally, recommended treatments should have been tested and then replicated in large, prospective, randomised, double-blind, controlled clinical trials by authorities in the field. For researcher residents, the persuasive strength of recommendations does not depend on where findings are published. Two doctors pointed out that the authoritative American Academy of Pediatrics regularly publishes guidelines that are not backed up with statistical evidence but only express the consensus of experts in the field. Such recommendations merely take the problem of basing medicine on routines to a professional level.

Researcher residents would not consider the parrot bite literature search an instance of EBM. Due to a small sample size, the evidence of rare conditions did not meet epidemiological norms but remained necessarily anecdotal. For researcher users of EBM, statistical criteria provide a gold standard for evaluating recommendations and while applying statistical measures, it is possible to make fine distinctions between studies. Researchers did not look in the scientific literature for pragmatic guidance to treat the patient at hand but for a variety of factors to take into consideration during decision-making.

Researchers struggled to make literature searches part of their daily practice. Because of the ease of access they frequently used MD Consult and review articles to keep abreast of the literature on common conditions. With rare conditions, however, many preferred to take the extra time to evaluate the primary literature and they frequented PubMed, Grateful Med, OVID, the Cochrane Library, and Medline. While researchers admitted that they might rely on a review article or a guideline for an on the spot dilemma, they acknowledged that they went back and assessed the literature more critically when they had the free time. Researchers stressed that the only way to keep in touch with the constant changes in medicine and provide the best clinical care was to continually keep up with the literature.

In sum, paediatric residents in both programmes reported that the use of evidence was actively encouraged and positively valued and that their involvement in EBM was inevitable. Yet, they defined EBM flexibly to match their own work approaches: librarians highlighted the practice of checking the literature when diagnostic or treatment problems arose. Researcher residents emphasised the scientific evaluation of research but they questioned the value of EBM's main instruments: clinical practice guidelines and research protocols.

Uncertainty and Evidence-Based Medicine

Sociological Scholarship

The concept of uncertainty plays a central role in medical sociology scholarship that addresses the question of how biomedical knowledge is acquired. Based on research conducted at the Cornell medical school during the early 1950s, Renée Fox argued that medical knowledge is inherently uncertain because it is riddled with gaps and unknowns and, secondly, because the amount of medical facts is ever-expanding and impossible to completely master (Fox 1957). The dilemma for students in medical school consists of managing the limitations of their own cognitive ability and the vast medical literature. During residents' clinical years, medical uncertainty emerges when students apply text knowledge to clinical situations and handle both the physiological and psychological aspects of patient care. Fox's sociology of knowledge consists of a gradual socialisation in medical confidence; instead of blaming oneself for clinical mistakes the aspiring doctor learns to successfully manage the limitations of medicine. Training for uncertainty serves to imprint a professional attitude of objective expertise and detached concern on the next generation of physicians. In later writings, Fox argued that uncertainty has become the hallmark of the entire field of medicine (Fox 2000). The recent influx of advanced medical technologies has created a sceptical attitude towards medicine's modernist promise to cure all, culminating in a culture of uncertainty.

Other authors have questioned the primacy of uncertainty and instead highlighted that 'training for control' closely follows 'training for uncertainty' (Atkinson 1984, Light 1979). Based on fieldwork among psychiatrists during their residency years, Donald Light for example, proposed that the goal of medical training is to teach young physicians how to control their uncertainties in order to become professional experts within their field (Light 1979). Light fine-tuned Fox's sources of clinical uncertainty in medical training and noted that aspiring physicians master medicine and gain control by 'psyching out' their instructors, limiting learning to relevant knowledge, acquiring clinical experience, focusing on technique, and gradually gaining autonomy. Light warns against an overconfident medical attitude centred in technique and disregarding patient-centred notions of health and illness.

While most sociologists – and also most medical practitioners – agree that the medical knowledge base is marred by various uncertainties, scholarly disagreements persist on the dominance of uncertainty and on whether uncertainty and certainty imply each other. Because EBM relies on a standardisation of medical knowledge and technique, it can be seen as a catalyst for these opposing viewpoints. In her most recent update of the uncertainty literature, Fox addresses the surge of EBM. Fox contends that EBM reinforces collective-oriented approaches in medicine at the expense of individualised patient–doctor interactions (Fox 2000). Siding with the critics of EBM, Fox remains apprehensive of EBM's narrow biomedical positivism and its threat to clinical expertise. Fox does not address the way EBM would impact medical socialisation but based on the central message of her earlier work, we would expect that the rise of EBM perpetuates scientific scepticism, a critical attitude of questioning evidence.

With Light we would expect that EBM brings about a dogmatic, control-centred form of medicine in resident's daily clinical practice, validating the power of medicine while accentuating the strengths and weaknesses of its scientific basis. Light notes that emphasising technique serves as a major form of professional control, providing a technical understanding of competence.

Research-Based Uncertainty

The residents we interviewed, however, noted that the most immediate effect of the increased reliance on guidelines or protocols and medical literature was a new source of uncertainty to be managed. Residents not only need to know how to diagnose and treat patients but need to acquire epidemiological research skills as well. Research-based uncertainty deals with the actual practice of conducting literature searches and evaluating studies. Even residents who rarely consulted primary research acknowledged that such critical assessment skills were expected of them. This form of uncertainty is closely aligned with the recent influx of information technologies and epidemiology in medicine. We found three instances of this novel uncertainty:

First, some residents felt uncomfortable about their ability to search for primary or review articles. Their concerns were focused on the skills required to effectively navigate the computer search engines. To conduct a good search, residents had to know which search engines existed, what kinds of information each source held, and how to search each one with appropriate key terms. Dr Cole described the difficulty he encountered when trying to master new search engines:

> [The library] has a number of other evidence-based programmes that I am not even familiar with, like the Cochrane data base and Best Evidence. I have tried to use them, but they are not so easy to just log-on and use. I have tried to just throw in a couple of terms, thinking it would be self-evident how it worked. It wasn't.

Not only the medical literature but also the databases keep changing. Secondly, librarians and researcher residents expressed similar doubts about their abilities to effectively evaluate a primary research article. Even Dr Mouton, who had worked for several years in biomedical research, acknowledged that she was 'not a very good statistician'. Other residents who had taken biostatistics or epidemiology courses, still felt unsure about their abilities to distinguish between a good and a bad sample, and statistical significance and confidence intervals.

Thirdly, residents questioned the interests behind conducting studies and expressed suspicion about effects of economical incentives on the quality of medical knowledge. Dr Weiss noted that: 'studies follow money, where money is, will be many studies. But at the same time, no one is going to do research on common things that we don't have any questions about'. The available research funding might thus sway the entire medical field. Paediatricians were particularly attuned to this inequity because comparatively little research exists on treatments and drug dosages for children.

The new research-based uncertainty leads to new forms of managing the uncertainty. Chief residents and attendings would organise journal clubs, where residents presented and critiqued articles, statistics refresher courses and tutorials on how to effectively use Medline. Guest speakers would tour departments and lecture on the primary research they had conducted. Learning how to deal with the specific uncertainty of research led, thus, to a new kind of research infused skill, an additional dimension of learning to doctor.

Does Managing Uncertainty Reinforce Dogmatism or Scepticism?

While earlier sociologists might have underestimated that a solution for dealing with uncertainty in itself creates new uncertainties that in turn call for new forms of uncertainty management, the issue at stake is the net result of the infusion of EBM: do residents display an attitude of scientific doubting as Fox predicted or does EBM confirm medical dogmatism as Light and others feared? The answer to that question depends on the different approaches of librarian and researcher residents towards the different sources of EBM. In short, librarians act more along the lines set out by Light while researchers follow Fox's predictions.

For librarians, practicing EBM with guidelines and review articles provided some comfort within the chaos of their clinical training. Residents suggested that a literature search allowed them to orient themselves when they had a diagnostic or a treatment question. They used the literature to make sure they were 'in the ballpark' before addressing the attending or their colleagues about a patient. Dr Cole gave an example of how EBM reduces clinical uncertainty. He talked about a patient with abnormal lab results possibly indicating hepatitis or myositis:

> People are still calling it a hepatitis/myositis, but I think that the only reason we are calling it hepatitis is because some of her liver function tests are abnormal, but it is only some of them and, it is the ones that could be elevated in skeletal–muscle disease. I think it is just going to be obvious to everyone when I tell them this afternoon. … I have these papers that say the [test results] can go up with skeletal–muscle disease. Boom! Now when I take it to them, I am more confident in my diagnosis.

The literature boosted Dr Cole's hunches. To find this type of comfort, however, librarian residents tended to search prepackaged EBM: review articles and guidelines where experts in the field had already sorted through the evidence. Dr McNair commented how a review article helped her determine the typical treatment for a diabetic child: 'I know a lot of pathophysiology, but I don't know how to do the work-up and treat the child. I use a lot of articles, especially review articles, large group studies, to figure out what my steps should be'.

Librarians mentioned that guidelines provided an additional kind of legal comfort that has become accentuated recently in North American health care. Dr McDougall explained the benefit: 'You always have clinical liability on your side. I follow the guidelines that the AAP has set. They can't fault you when you have done everything you can for that person'. In contrast, consulting clinical trials might present legal pitfalls. Dr Tomassi warned:

> A lot of times the primary literature is very much like 'well some studies suggest this, some studies suggest that' and then you don't know what the hell to do with this. Do I want to do anything because I read it in an article that I am not familiar with? Will that get me sued or kill a patient because just some study told me so?

Researchers, however, were hesitant about using the authority of guidelines to make themselves feel more comfortable or to provide legal protections. Dr Mouton suggested that guidelines might make residents feel too complacent:

> One of the things that I think is wrong is if you go into medical school and grasp whatever bit of guidelines you can get to cover your insecurities. If you do that than you stop thinking. People stop using their common sense. [A guideline] doesn't mean that you shouldn't examine the baby.

To avoid a false sense of security, researchers tended to critically question the directives of guidelines and review articles instead of taking it as medical gospel.

With clinical trials and other forms of primary research, the opinions ran opposite. Librarian researcher residents remarked that primary studies inevitably generated contradictions and confusions. Dr Fletcher stressed her frustration:

> This is probably a little too honest. But you spend all this time reading that stinking study and then you come up with one thing at the very end. The result was maybe this or maybe that. And sometimes it is equivocal. [She throws up her arms.] I just want to know what is done. What is the result?

Dr Mouton, more of a researcher, stressed instead that the contradictions revealed in primary research do not necessarily lead to worse clinical practice. She stated:

> It is very hard to find certain truths. The literature doesn't help you to find those kinds of securities. The literature makes you aware of all the little edges. When you go to the literature you always find something that makes you think: 'Oh, I shouldn't forget that'. When you do a literature search it makes you more knowledgeable. Being more knowledgeable makes you more certain where you stand.

While for librarians the primary literature perpetuated confusion and led to an avoidance of such studies, researchers acknowledged the conflicting picture of different studies and stressed – in Dr Mouton's words – that 'controversy is part of life, part of research, part of science'. Primary research alerted researcher residents to factors and variations of clinical practice that they should not take for granted. The result was a more complex decision-making process in which uncertainties within medical knowledge were incorporated.

When applying EBM to clinical dilemmas they face in their practice, librarians and researchers were again at odds about the merits of evidence. For librarians, any literature search was fundamentally incomplete. Dr Tomassi put the problem simply: 'Guidelines cannot diagnose the patient for me'. Librarians reacted against the widespread perception that EBM would take the place of clinical judgment, reducing them to mere short-order cooks who followed 'cookbook-recipe' medicine. For librarians, the ultimate litmus test of reducing uncertainty and gaining certitude is having done things repeatedly in the past, that is, accumulating clinical judgment. Whether such judgment was grounded in the 'attending's standard of care' or in the literature did not matter much. Because the attending's advice was likely to be tailored to the individual patient's situation, it might have an edge for residents in training. One resident noted that he seemed to get clinical results, regardless of the source he used. And if he did not obtain expected results, he would try something different the next time. This philosophy led librarian residents to avoid doing too many literature searches.

Researcher residents were also aware of the gap between the literature and clinical practice in the immediate pressures of residency life. Dr Weiss articulated the tensions:

> The limitations (of EBM) are that it is tough to access unless you have the time to do it all the time … unless you are really up on the literature. It is kind of like surfing. Once you are on the board and going down the wave it is easy; but you have to paddle and get up on the board first. I guess as a resident you are too busy just trying to make sure the board doesn't come crashing down on you to do that.

But where librarians considered literature searches, at best, a dubious tool for reducing clinical uncertainty and more commonly a source of extra frustration, researchers embraced dealing with the contradictions and confounding variables of both patient care and the literature as real medical work. Teasing out protocols and research findings was as important as managing blood pressure. One of the surprising findings in our interviews was that the clinical examples provided by the most EBM knowledgeable residents centred on disregarding research, adapting protocols and guidelines, or filling gaps in the literature. Researchers argued that EBM might lead to better physicians who know when not to follow research-based guidelines and recommendations. For example, Dr Morris told us that in a paediatric resuscitation she had ordered the nurses to give the sodium bicarbonate drug all at once instead of giving it at time intervals as the Advanced Cardiac Life Support protocol recommended.

In conclusion, librarians look to the research literature for ready answers but are disappointed with the uncertainty inherent in medical knowledge. Researchers, on the other hand, trust that uncertainty produced by the literature and clinical practice creates a positive flux of increased knowledge. Librarian's instrumentalist use of the literature is more likely to confirm a dogmatic clinical practice. Librarians might overstate the certainty of research and take recommendations at face value, or – more commonly – they might get frustrated with the residual uncertainty of research findings and avoid researching altogether. Researchers approach the literature from a more relativist perspective. They do not expect clear answers but a sharpening of discriminatory power that will aid them in patient decision-making. Researchers apply the critical assessment skills touted by EBM advocates to EBM itself, leading to a sceptical research attitude and disregarding of EBM. Fox's analysis seems thus to be more geared towards a minority group of researcher residents who adopt uncertainty as their clinical *leitmotiv* while Light quite accurately predicted the attitude of librarians for whom the urge to dominate clinical uncertainty with readymade knowledge prevails.

EBM and the Humanitarian Critique

None of these scholars, however, predicted the counterintuitive extent to which the turn to standardised techniques might actually validate humanitarian medicine. Within the sociological discussion of uncertainty resides a strong critique that technological values and incentives push medicine to abandon open-minded, holistic caring for patients. The science of biomedicine threatens the art of caring. Standardisation leads to technological hubris – overconfidence at the expense of appropriate patient care. For Fox, the culture of uncertainty spawns ethical dilemmas and ambivalence in medicine. The issue about uncertainty is not even whether doctors know enough to heal but, more profoundly, whether physicians truly have the interest of their patients in mind (Fox 2000). According to Light, the turn away from caring is fuelled by medicine's inability to deal with uncertainty and urge to over-control. Physicians seek refuge in techniques to sidestep more confounding issues about equity, pain, grief, and patient satisfaction.

Neither librarians nor researchers expressed an abandonment of humanitarian values due to EBM. Librarian's tendency for dogmatism with regard to literature findings did not extend to their attitude toward patients. Librarians generally rejected a technological or scientistic mindset and instead highlighted the importance of being attuned to patient needs. Dr Fletcher, for example, ran a laboratory test with little hope that it would get at the root of a patient's obesity because testing would appease the patient's mother. Researchers' critical assessment of the literature resulted in questioning the strength of any research recommendation and often also in disregarding or adapting recommendations. As a result, researchers reported to opt for less aggressive care (for example, not to over-prescribe antibiotics), a stronger emphasis on listening and observing patients, and even paying attention to one's 'gut feeling'.

The residents largely interpreted the perceived shortcomings of EBM as redemption of clinical judgment. Research did not constitute a final technologised directive but at best a suggestion to be evaluated with a patient in mind (Timmermans and Berg 1997, 2003). Senior resident Dr Brown articulated this idea: 'The real uncertainty comes at the end of the day when you're at home thinking "did I do the right thing?" or "did I not do the right thing?". That is not when you are having Medline at the corner of your eye'. Dr Brown added: 'A lot of medicine is dealing with social, psychological, emotional stuff that impacts the physical and there is not much literature about that. That is not something you can read about, that is something you have to learn and do'. Based on residents' own assessment, EBM leads thus paradoxically to a re-appreciation of clinical judgment and listening to patients.

The Social Context of EBM and the Politics of Uncertainty

Forging a tight link between knowledge and power, EBM advocates also promise a new meritocratic political order on the hospital ward: power differences should be based on familiarity with the literature instead of institutionalised seniority. New residents of a San Francisco hospital, for example, receive a written manifesto about EBM. Evidence 'levels the intellectual playing field: Everyone's clinical opinion counts equally, regardless of rank or experience. We value opinions only to the extent that they are supported by scientific evidence' (Grimes 1995: 453).

The democratisation impetus of EBM should take away an important source of uncertainty during medical socialisation. Because of the vagueness of evaluation criteria during medical training, residents constantly wonder what their instructors are looking for. The solution to this problem in the past has been to 'psych out' instructors by asking them directly what they want and by observing them to infer expectations (Becker et al. 1961, Light 1979). EBM might take the guess work out of the education process and at the same time subvert the power relationships away from local conformity, requiring a revision of this aspect of the socialisation scholarship.

Regardless of whether they used the literature as researchers or librarians, the respondents strongly emphasised that EBM has not democratised the resident–attending relationship. The reality of the paediatric residency training is that most residents only in emergency situations decide upon their own treatments without previously consulting a senior resident or attending. Within a supervisory apprenticeship, the aim of residency is to build a foundation in a variety of paediatric cases. Dr Weiss explained:

The idea of residency is to get in there first, find out what your gut feeling is, what you think it is, and then present it to somebody else and bounce it off them. They will say, 'I disagree with this. You forgot this. You might want to look into this'.

Almost all examples of medical decision-making provided by the residents included checking ideas with senior residents or attendings.

As a consequence, residents denied an increase in knowledge-based egalitarianism. Dr Mouton acknowledged that regardless of her familiarity with the literature she was 'the lowest on the whole ladder here'. Dr Abraham added, 'I don't feel like I am on the same level with anybody right now'. Because residents reside at the bottom of a steep authority ladder, few residents actively challenged attendings or pointed out that their superior's recommendations were outdated even when their own critical literature and research review suggested alternative patient management. At best they might engage in a polite, face-saving discussion about what might be most beneficial for the patient or ask the attending what they thought of a particular alternative. Even in such exchanges when residents cautiously questioned an attending based on evidence from the literature, most residents reported that they and the literature would likely lose out. Dr Wilson noted that 'at those times it tends to fall back on experience. [The attending would say:] "Well that may work, but I have seen in this case, this works better. So we are going this way"'. The attending would qualify the study's findings with some reason why the recommendations did not apply in this particular case.

Residents noted that they were unlikely to know as much about the patient or the literature, and that they lacked the 30 years of experience to engage in a discussion among equals. The attending was not only likely to have more experience with patients but, particularly in teaching hospitals, were likely to keep up with the literature. In addition, the attending might have inside knowledge to qualify the reading such as the reputation of a particular hospital for orthopaedics, the extent to which a particular author opts for unnecessary tests, or the kind of publishing criteria used in a particular journal.

Despite the lack of democratisation with science, EBM impacted the relationship between attendings and residents because it restructured the knowledge exchange. EBM offered residents and attendings an external criterion to evaluate the knowledge base of the other. In contrast to their image in the EBM literature, most attendings are not keepers of outdated traditions but instead guarantors of EBM usage, ensuring continuous reminders and consistency (Latour 1999). EBM became integrated in a hierarchical relationship where superiors asked residents to conduct literature searches when questions arose. Dr Wilson explained: 'it is not uncommon to have your attending ask you, "why don't you check that out?" or "why don't you see if you can find some information about that"'. Once the resident comes up with the most recent literature, an attending might sit down with them and discuss the strengths and weaknesses of the evidence.

When residents encounter a dilemma or new situation, a literature review allows them to channel their ignorance before they approach the attending. Dr Weiss put it this way, 'Guidelines ensure that you are not totally in left field. It gives you a chance of not missing something that you shouldn't have missed, but you don't have the experience to know that yet. So, it buys you somebody else's experience, I guess'. The protocols and research recommendations gave the resident a hunch of what this patient might be all about but whether clues translated into realities depended on whether the attending would go along with the recommendations or instead suggest alternatives. It was often simpler and easier to ask than to research.

Attendings and residents who take EBM's democratisation promise seriously are thus in for a rude awakening. Residents overwhelmingly acknowledged that even with clinical practice guidelines and research protocols hierarchy differences are real and cannot be ignored. Attendings function not only as more experienced colleagues but also as supervisors whose evaluations carry much weight. Even when protocols and guidelines spell out best practices, residents still need to decipher – in Dr Chambliss's words – 'the attending's best practice'. The influx of EBM thus does not require a revision of the power differences in the sociological socialisation literature. This does not mean that EBM has no political effects in medical training: within the context of the resident–attending relationship, EBM forms an external validation criterion for both resident and attending to check the other's knowledge base. In light of these changes, Dr Rosenberg granted that instead of levelling the playing field, EBM 'brings the field a little bit closer'.

Evidence-Based Clinical Judgment

Wherever we turn, EBM seems to run into a barrier of clinical judgment and experience. Research-based knowledge seems to perpetually fall short in clinical decision making. Residents refer to the extra quality needed as 'experience', 'competence', or 'confidence'. Sociologists seem to agree with medical practitioners when they stress that control over uncertainty is achieved with a growing sense of confidence. Concepts such as confidence, certitude, and experience are crucial in socialisation theory, but they remain difficult to articulate and most sociologists attribute experience simply to the resident's seniority (Fox 1957, Merton, Reader and Kendall 1957). After some time, the resident somehow has acquired experience and gained confidence. Part of the conceptual difficulty is that experience and evidence continue to be viewed as distinct, and even opposite entities.

Residents' encounters with EBM show that the opposition between experience and evidence is false. Any consultation of written research is already pre-structured by the overall diagnostic or treatment goal and informed by other research and accumulated clinical observations. Similarly, any experience is grounded in the hierarchy of written research evidence, anecdotes, consensus and hunches of generations of clinicians and basic researchers. Evidence and experience constitute complimentary resources that help residents in learning treatment options and patient management (Freidson 1986). The point of EBM in residency training is not to impose simplistic rule following but to offer a justification for clinical decision making. As we have seen, librarians will check ready-made evidence while researchers are more likely to assess primary literature. But those findings are filtered through the attending who, in turn, has accumulated an amalgam of patient experiences and research findings. The quality that guides clinical decision-making is then not the tradition bound experience put up as a straw person in the medical and sociological literature but a mixture of skills and uncertainties grounded in medical knowledge that could be more accurately called evidence-based clinical judgment.

Evidence-based clinical judgment has several important characteristics. First, it cannot be reduced to either evidence or experience but contains inevitably a mixture of the two, albeit not necessarily in equal proportions. Librarians as a group tend to prefer the hands-on handling of patients and the visual instruction of attendings while researcher residents ground their expertise in the literature. But librarians still need to acquire evidence to back up their practice while researchers fall back on hands-on patient handling to decide how the literature applies. Second, residents exhibiting good evidence-based clinical judgment do not necessarily use more literature but exhibit an awareness of all the factors necessary to reach a satisfactory medical decision. A competent resident knows when literature reviews will likely lead to better patient care, how to evaluate research findings effectively, how to check the findings with the attending in a way that preserves the senior's authority, and how to communicate the proposed decision plan with the patient to ensure adequate compliance. Evidence-based clinical judgment includes thus epidemiological and social skills. Third, it also is not a quality that residents aspire and attendings possess. Both act based on evidence-based clinical judgment. The difference between residents and attendings is not simply a matter of seniority or more hands-on work but is also influenced by the scope of their responsibility and their institutionalised power advantage. Fourth, evidence-based clinical judgment is part of the process of managing uncertainties during residency training. Evidence-based judgement evolves as new contingencies in patient care crop up, when mistakes are made, or when previous recommendations are reconsidered. Finally, evidence-based clinical judgment is ultimately grounded in a western allopathic, and professionalised approach to medicine.

Although rooted in research and literature, evidence-based clinical judgment moves the resident away from a strict interpretation of the literature. A physician starts with a recommendation and adds qualifications to consider whether the guideline applies to this particular patient, ward, attending, time-frame, and resources. The generation of evidence-based clinical judgment allows residents to apply protocols to patients for whom it was not intended because they gained insights into the rationale behind the evidence. It also facilitates skipping or substituting steps, working around the protocols, and appropriating them. The resident interacts with the protocols and guidelines. More than the mere passing of time, the relative value of factors to be taken into consideration marks the accumulation of evidence-based clinical judgment.

Conclusion

Evidence-based medicine is everywhere in contemporary health care. In one decade, the number of articles in Pubmed with evidence-based medicine as a MeSH term increased seven-fold with a total of more than 30,000 articles over the decade. It is difficult to argue with the basic premise that health care interventions should be based on scientific evidence. Still, social scientists have questioned whether RCTs constitute the best possible evidence under all circumstances and whether standardisation will lead to better clinical care (Grossman and MacKenzie 2005, Lambert 2006, Timmermans and Berg 2003). They have, in turn, situated the emergence of EBM as a professional strategy to offset the likelihood of reforms enforced by government agencies and insurance companies (Denny 1999, Pope 2003, Rappolt 1997, Timmermans and Kolker 2004, Traynor 2000). EBM is embraced as a solution for the problem of practice variation due to physicians following traditional authority or anecdote. An industry of conducting RCTs and reviewing evidence in consensus conferences and specialised organisations helped disseminate EBM across the medical spectrum. As the experience in medical education shows, however, it is unclear what the actual effect is of EBM on the behaviour of clinicians. While EBM may have sensitised the current generation of health care providers to research methodology and epidemiology, logistical and cognitive barriers have created an implementation gap in medical decision making. In the ongoing struggles between medical sub disciplines and between alternative and allopathic medicine (Barry 2006, Borgerson 2005), the commodification of the pharmaceutical industry (Greene 2007) and the power hierarchy of medical schools, EBM has not infused medicine with scientific rationality but has been mobilised as a political tool to stake out an advantageous position.

An examination of how medical students practice medicine in an EBM-infused environment constitutes a call for examining what actually happened rather than what would hypothetically happen if EBM was implemented. As the discussion between researchers and librarians hinted at, even among health care providers EBM is many things to many people: everyone seems to be doing EBM but tremendous differences exist in how clinicians engage with evidence. Within the social science literature, the absence of patient perspectives is glaring, although some social scientists have advanced theoretical arguments about the kind of experiences that patients can bring up in an EBM-infused care context (May et al. 2006). Most of the EBM literature still follows a professional extract and apply approach to patient relationships in which clinicians view patients as objects of information gathering, care providers make decisions, and the presumption is that the actual patient relationship does not change but that patients simply receive better care (Upshur 2005). With clinical practice guidelines only a website away, direct-to-consumer advertising, and vocal patient health movements actively involved in the production of scientific knowledge (Epstein 1997), the patient–provider relationship under EBM is likely more dialogical and complicated. In fact, patient preferences are often cited as a reason for the EBM implementation gap (Upshur 2005).

What, then, is the effect of a broadly supported standardisation movement for residents' work? While critics consider guidelines and protocols one more nail in the coffin of humanised health care and advocates hail standardisation as the means to render medicine scientific, we notice a more moderate effect. Protocols and guidelines do not replace but reorient judgment. EBM allows residents to approach attendings and patients with comfort in certain circumstances and with renewed trepidation (because the literature is not conclusive or unequivocal) in other situations. The influx of EBM shifts residents' attention to a more elaborate set of biomedical and epidemiological variables.

Yet, it would be wrong to conclude that such a reorientation renders medicine less humanistic or diminishes residents' faith in the overall purpose of medicine. If the research on uncertainty validates any functionalist premise, it is the premise of unintended consequences. New medical technologies might as well lead to increased choice, access, equity, and patient autonomy as to objectification, overspecialisation, and bureaucratisation. Managing uncertainty similarly has a myriad of consequences that cannot be decided *a priori*. Our research suggests that the perceived inadequacy of available evidence might lead to a validation of humanistic concerns.

In sum, our retooling of the uncertainty concept in light of EBM centres it in the sociology of knowledge and technology. Our conclusion is that EBM's standardisation urge did neither eradicate nor reinforce but transformed uncertain medical knowledge. EBM's legacy crystallises in the honing of evidence-based clinical judgment and is as apparent in disregarding and avoiding research as it is in protocol following and routine research consultations.

Acknowledgements

This chapter is a revised and updated version of an article published in the *Journal of Health and Social Behavior*, 42(4), 2001. Permission no: 005734 from the American Sociological Association.

References

Atkinson, P. 1984. Training for certainty. *Social Science and Medicine*, 19(9), 949–56.
Barry, C. 2006. The role of evidence in alternative medicine: Contrasting biomedical and anthropological approaches. *Social Science and Medicine*, 62(11), 2646–57.

Bazarian, J., Davis, C., Spillane, L., Blumstein, H. and Schneider, S. 1999. Teaching emergency medicine residents evidence-based critical appraisal skills: A controlled trial. *Annals of Emergency Medicine*, 34(2), 148–54.

Becker, H., Geer, B., Hughes, E. and Strauss, A. 1961. *Boys in White: Student Culture in Medical School*. Chicago: University of Chicago Press.

Borgerson, K. 2005. Evidence-based alternative medicine? *Perspectives in Biology and Medicine*, 48(4), 502–15.

Denny, K. 1999. Evidence-based medicine and medical authority. *Journal of Medical Humanities*, 20(4), 247–63.

Eisenberg, J. 1999. Ten lessons for evidence-based technology assessment. *JAMA: The Journal of the American Medical Association*, 282(19), 1865–9.

Epstein, S. 1997. Activism, drug regulation, and the politics of therapeutic evaluating in the AIDS era: A case study of ddC and the 'surrogate markers' debate. *Social Studies of Science*, 27(5), 691–726.

Foucault, M. 1973. *The Birth of the Clinic*. New York: Vintage Books.

Fox, R. 1957. Training for uncertainty, in *The Student Physician*, edited by R. Merton, G. Reader and P. Kendall. Cambridge: Harvard University Press.

Fox, R. 2000. Medical uncertainty revisited, in *The Handbook of Social Studies in Health and Medicine*, edited by G. Albrecht, R. Fitzpatrick and S. Scrimshaw. London: SAGE Publications.

Freidson, E. 1986. *Professional Powers: A Study of the Institutionalization of Formal Knowledge*. Chicago: Chicago University Press.

Friedland, D. 1999. *Evidence Based Medicine: A Framework for Clinical Practice*. Connecticut: Appleton and Lange.

Ghali, W., Saitz, R., Eskew, A., Gupta, M., Quan, H. and Hershman, W. 2000. Successful teaching in evidence-based medicine. *Medical Education*, 34(1), 18–22.

Good, M. 1998. *American Medicine: The Quest for Competence*. Berkeley: California University Press.

Graef, J. 1997. *Manual of Pediatric Therapeutics*. Philadelphia: Lippinscott Raven.

Greene, J. 2007. *Prescribing by Numbers*. Baltimore: Johns Hopkins University Press.

Grimes, D. 1995. Introducing evidence-based medicine into a department of obstetrics and gynecology. *Obstetrics and Gynecology*, 86(3), 451–7.

Grossman, J. and Mackenzie, F. 2005. The randomized controlled trial: Gold standard or merely standard. *Perspectives in Biology and Medicine*, 48(4), 516–34.

Hafferty, F. 2000. Reconfiguring the sociology of medical education: Emerging topics and pressing issues, in *Handbook of Medical Sociology*, 5th edition, edited by C. Bird, P. Conrad and A. Fremont. New Jersey: Prentice Hall.

Lambert, H. 2006. Accounting for EBM: Notions of evidence in medicine. *Social Science and Medicine*, 62(11), 2633–45.

Latour, B. 1999. *Pandora's Hope: Essays on the Reality of Science Studies.* Cambridge: Harvard University Press.

Light, D. 1979. Uncertainty and control in professional training. *Journal of Health and Social Behavior*, 20(4), 310–22.

May, C., Rapley, T., Moreira, T., Finch, T. and Heaven, B. 2006. Technogovernance: Evidence, subjectivity, and the clinical encounter in primary care medicine. *Social Science and Medicine*, 62(4), 1022–30.

Merton, R., Reader, G. and Kendall, P. 1957. *The Student-Physician: Introductory Studies in the Sociology of Medical Education.* Cambridge: Harvard University Press for the Commonwealth Fund.

Pope, C. 2003. Resisting evidence: The study of evidence-based medicine as a contemporary social movement. *Health*, 7(3), 267–82.

Rappolt, S. 1997. Clinical guidelines and the fate of medical autonomy in Ontario. *Social Science and Medicine*, 44(7), 977–87.

Siberry, G. and Iannone, R. (eds). 2000. *The Harriet Lane Handbook: A Manual for Pediatric House Officers.* St. Louis: Mosby.

Starr, P. 1982. *The Social Transformation of Medicine.* New York: Basic Books.

Strauss, A. 1987. *Qualitative Analysis for Social Scientists.* Cambridge: Cambridge University Press.

Timmermans, S. and Berg, M. 1997. Standardization in action: Achieving local universality through medical protocols. *Social Studies of Science*, 27(2), 769–99.

Timmermans, S. and Berg, M. 2003. *The Gold Standard: The Challenge of Evidence-Based Medicine and Standardization in Health Care.* Philadelphia: Temple University Press.

Timmermans, S. and Kolker, E. 2004. Evidence-based medicine and the reconfiguration of medical knowledge. *Journal of Health and Social Behavior*, 45, 177–93.

Traynor, M. 2000. Purity, conversion and the evidence-based movements. *Health*, 4(2), 139–58.

Upshur, R. 2005. Looking for rules in a world of exceptions. *Perpectives in Biology and Medicine*, 48(4), 477–89.

Chapter 3

Resisting Stratification: Imperialism, War Machines and Evidence-Based Practice

Dave Holmes and Patrick O'Byrne

Introduction

Within the health care disciplines, the topic and idea of evidence-based practice has become a major point of discussion and contention. This debate has arisen, in part, because patients want to be reassured that the procedures and treatments which clinicians recommend and perform are both research-based and likely to produce their intended outcomes. Simultaneously, clinicians want to know that the information they relay is accurate and that the practices they undertake consistently produce their planned effects. Lastly, health care funders (whether tax payers in public systems or insurance companies in private systems) want to ensure that their monetary investments will yield tangible outcomes; is money being spent on efficacious and effective procedures and interventions? From the perspective of these three stakeholders (patients, practitioners and payers), evidence-based practice is surely beneficial. It is a much-needed response to the traditional approach that has and continues to pervade many areas of health care: that is, evidence-based practice contrasts with the strategy of basing health care service delivery solely on anecdotal evidence or on the 'it has always been done like this' mentality.

However, the foregoing points do not make evidence-based practice exempt from critique. There is still a need for an attitude of caution regarding this approach because, while the idea that health care should be supported by evidence is sound, evidence-based practice does not exclusively denote the use of evidence in practice. Instead, it is a philosophy for understanding and approaching practice, evidence and research. It is a perspective wherein certain knowledge development strategies are afforded greater prestige and position, and by extension, so are the corresponding data that these methods generate (Holmes et al. 2006a). The converse is also true: certain research designs, data collection and analysis strategies, and paradigmatic perspectives are relegated to inferior positions. Evidence-based practice thus entails a ranking and sorting of evidence and research design – a process that its proponents often declare is warranted because the allegedly inferior approaches (such as qualitative observation and/or interview) do not produce sufficiently robust evidence to guarantee the delivery of health care services in appropriate and consistent ways (Holmes et al. 2008).

The examination of evidence-based practice that is endorsed herein, however, is not an outright rejection of evidence or its use in health care practice or service delivery. Similarly, the critique that is recommended is not a simple commentary regarding the status of certain research designs, such as the acceptance of randomised controlled trials as the research gold standard. We acknowledge, for example, that evidence-based practitioners have adopted an array of context-specific gold standards: randomised controlled trials only assume this position in intervention studies; by comparison, cohort studies are often the gold standard in aetiological research. Moreover, as researchers and clinicians ourselves, we both strive to develop and utilise evidence in our daily work.

Consequently, we reject neither the idea of evidence, nor that of evidence-based practice. What we wish to put forth, instead, is a sociopolitical examination about the state and nature of an approach to health care that can be succinctly summarised as a systematisation of knowledge within a post-positivistic epistemology. What we aim to undertake is an analysis about the gold standard phenomenon itself. We advocate for investigations into the social parameters that permit such statements as gold standard to even make sense. Accordingly, we suggest that questions should be asked about the principles that underpin this approach to health care practice (whether clinical, policy-based or administrative). For one, how can we understand the situation that is evidence-based practice?

To answer this question we will employ the works of Michel Foucault, Gilles Deleuze, Felix Guattari, Michael Hardt and Antonio Negri. Specifically, we will invoke Foucault's ideas about power/knowledge, Deleuze-Guattari's writings on stratification and the war machine(resistance) and Hardt-Negri's work on empire. In combination, this work will be used to suggest that, as a distinct phenomenon, evidence-based practice is a form of stratification – a strategy of sorting and ranking evidence, research designs *et cetera* that seems to be in everyone's best interests (such as patients, the public, clinicians, policy-makers and funders). As part of examining this process, we will also argue that evidence-based practice, in its current form, is a political process.

In building these arguments, we will demonstrate that, to date, evidence-based practice has progressed through two main waves. The first, an exclusionary phase, was a period when evidence-based practice proponents rejected nearly all forms of evidence that were not quantitative or epidemiological in nature. In this first phase, not only were hardly any research designs accepted/acceptable, but also most non-quantitative data collection techniques were routinely rejected (see, for example, Davidoff et al. 1995). This means that evidence-based practice was based almost exclusively on numerical measurements. Since this time, however, a second wave has arisen, and it has expanded the reductive character of the biomedical hierarchy of evidence and the domination of experimental/epidemiological design strategies therein that characterised evidence-based practice's first wave. This new phase, by comparison, is much more inclusive of non-quantitative research techniques.

However, this new phase in the history of evidence-based practice (in which many forms of evidence and data collection are now deemed acceptable) carries an important caveat: while the evidence-based practice approach has undeniably become more inclusive, there still exists a hesitation toward, and subordination of, many of the newly accepted forms of data collection. A powerful, post-positivistic-based systemisation of care continues to pervade evidence-based practice.

Consequently, while the evidence-based way of seeing and being in the world seems to promote the idea of using best knowledge to produce best practices (which is assumed to be a process that is free of political bias), this line of thinking silently enforces specific research designs and worldviews by implying that some knowledge is inherently better than others (Holmes, Roy and Perron 2008). It is argued here that the Cochrane taxonomy (a well-known example of a codified system for ranking evidence and knowledge; Cochrane Consumer Network 2010) functions as one such a political device, not as a scientific tool. It is an imperial apparatus of capture (that will be explained shortly in its Deleuzo-Guattarian/Hardt-Negrian sense), which ranks the methods of knowledge development and relegates certain approaches to inferior positions. In other words, the second wave of evidence-based practice exemplifies the techniques which are described by Hardt-Negri's definition of empire. In opposition to the violence of this stratification we suggest that a Deleuzo-Guattarian war machine, which symbolises resistance, is needed. Indeed, we need to deconstruct the contemporary systemisation of care that occurs within the health care approach known as evidence-based practice.

Epistemè: Evidence-Based Practice as a Way of Thinking

To begin, we ground our discussion by using the concept of *epistemè* (from the Greek word meaning 'worldview'). We start in this way because we wish to describe the sociopolitical factors that render evidence-based practice (and all of its corresponding terminology and ideas) knowable and an *epistemè* describes the accepted or dominant manner of gaining and organising knowledge in a given period. In short, *epistemès* inform people's ways of seeing and knowing the world (Holmes et al. 2008). To continue, an *epistemè* is the implicit basis for knowledge, the condition of possibility for something to appear to people as true or false, good or bad (Foucault 1997). We believe that evidence-based practice is a component of the contemporary health sciences *epistemè*, a relationship which makes this concept an appropriate starting point for discussing evidence-based practice. Indeed, a concept that describes a strategic apparatus that operates covertly and which underpins people's comprehension of the world is ideal for understanding the phenomenon that is evidence-based practice.

Dominating/dominant *epistemès* are expressed through institutions, such as healthcare settings, and through specific disciplines, such as medicine or nursing (Holmes et al. 2008). Despite the widespread nature of *epistemè*, it is difficult if not impossible to see how a specific *episteme* frames one's perceptions; it comprises governing rules and ideologies, but they are rarely codified or acknowledged in an overt and identifiable manner (Foucault 1997, Murray, Holmes and Rail 2008). Consequently, one can only recognie *episteme* by virtue of their effects – that is, by describing, analysing and discussing that which structures social interactions, guides interpersonal connection and organises both individual and group behaviour. By engaging in such analyses *episteme* become visible (Foucault 1997).

A recent example of an *episteme* is the early twentieth century eugenic discourse about healthy nations. The effect of this discourse was, in part, based on an *episteme* 'that informed a science of race, purity, intelligence, disease and so forth' (Holmes et al. 2008: 396). However, because *episteme* are hidden within the assumptions that help give meaning to ideas and actions, a definition of these systems can only emerge by means of in-depth analysis.

Epistemès and their effects are intricate and far-reaching. As such, they drive specific actions, allow for (or ban) knowledge development in certain areas and foster the development and implementation of regulatory mechanisms in particular ways. The pervasiveness of *epistemès* is also evident in the fact that these apparatuses are supported by a myriad of interconnected institutions and disciplines, many of which co-operatively, but often unknowingly, function to maintain specific constructions of reality (Foucault 1997, Holmes et al. 2008). Take, for instance, the collusion that can occur between various organisations (such as universities, funding agencies and professional bodies) regarding the use of evidence-based practice principles in research, education and clinical practice (Holmes et al. 2006a).

This often-unintentional collaboration typically occurs because different groups, with varying degrees of social authority, such as physicians, nurses and the schools that educate these health professionals, believe and proclaim that they investigate and seek objective knowledge. However, it is just as likely that the members of these groups are measuring 'epistemic compliance' (Holmes et al. 2008: 396). That is, the members of these professions and education institutions determine how consistent new information is with that which is already known. The (perhaps unintentional but nevertheless achieved) outcome of this sequence is that the *status quo* system of social dominance continues.[1]

The evidence-based practice movement is therefore a defining feature of the contemporary health sciences *episteme*, as can be seen in the language that its proponents use to describe this paradigmatically positivistic systemisation of

---

1   This maintenance of social dominance should not be interpreted in a Marxist sense; rather, a Deleuzo-Guattarian interpretation, particularly one that revolves around the concept of microfascism should be used to understand this claim. According to this concept, everyone is complicit in social, political and knowledge-based hierarchies. In relation to evidence-based practice, it may be the quantitative researchers who purport their research to be best, but it is also the qualitative researchers who complacently allow such claims to stand unchallenged.

care. For example, Davidoff and colleagues (1995: 1085), in an early editorial on evidence-based practice in the *British Medical Journal*, provided the following description about what constitutes evidence: 'In essence, evidence-based medicine is rooted in ... identifying the best evidence [which] means using epidemiological and bio-statistical ways of thinking'. The language used in this quotation is important because 'it constitutes not just ways of speaking rhetorically, but ways of thinking epistemically, and ultimately, ways of being in the world, ontologically' (Holmes et al. 2008: 396). As a part of the construction, articulation and perpetuation of the *epistemè* that enables evidence-based practice to make sense, there has been a corresponding 'proliferation of specialised jargon, conferences, university curricula, journals and so forth' (Holmes et al. 2008: 396). This, in turn, has led to an increased mobilisation of resources and the implementation of many evidence-based practice interventions – all of which have further supported the hegemonic influence of this movement. One possible outcome of this process is the construction of a 'self-maintaining and self-fulfilling phenomenon' that increasingly ranks evidence on one hand, and which gains more prestige, power and social acceptance as a result of this proliferation on the other hand (Holmes et al. 2008: 396).

Evidence-based practice, therefore, is a fundamental aspect of the current health sciences *epistemè*, a political mechanism that has pervaded scientific investigation and which is evident because of its specialised vocabulary, institutions and advocates. Indeed, evidence-based practice characterises the contemporary health services *epistemé* because it is the dominant framework within which statements, ideas and opinions can be understood. In short, it is the system within which thought and behaviour make sense and become knowable (Holmes et al. 2006a, 2006b).

The First Wave of Evidence-Based Practice: Stratification and Politics

To further explore evidence-based practice and how it operates as a dominant *epistemè* in contemporary health sciences work, we now draw on Deleuze and Guattari's (1987) concept of stratification. The benefit of using this idea is that it helps to situate how knowledge, knowledge development and the *epistemè* within which such processes operate are techniques for fixedly organising (stratifying) often disparate, but nevertheless interrelated, occurrences, technologies, artefacts and phenomena. Evidence-based practice, as such, is a method of stratification that corresponds with the post-enlightenment idea of searching for the one true answer, the one right way of understanding and the one best method for practising clinically. Evidence-based practice is thus both a form of stratification (that is, a ranking and sorting process itself) and the outcome of a certain form of stratification (known as the overarching *epistemè*).

To explain further, stratification is a method of allotting specific phenomena not just to, but also into, designed locations, either temporarily or permanently

(May 2005). It is a term which describes the processes of fixed designation and distribution and it is the underpinning of *epistemè*: the rules of *epistemè* permit specific facets of a generalised whole to be extracted and linked together in such a way that only certain identifiable outcomes are possible. Stated differently, *epistemè* ensure that only certain outcomes are understandable; all others seem to be nonsensical. Stratification, as an integral part of this process, is the operation of labelling observations cogently and assigning objects to specific locations based on preconceived ideations about the world (Deleuze and Guattari 1987). The outcome is a pseudo-Cartesian mapping of both physical and non-physical space: the act of assigning relative positions, of identifying that which constitutes normal or abnormal, and, in this case, of ranking knowledge and its various methods of development. This, as just noted, occurs based on already-established rules about what is possible, about what is allowable and about who is able to make such declarations/assertions – it is the outcome of epistemic directives, that is.

According to Deleuze and Guattari, such stratification maintains that only certain people are allowed to speak in critical forums and that they are only allowed to do so if they speak in an appropriate fashion about acceptable topics. For example, in the evidence-based practice domain, only clinicians who are armed with certain information are allowed to speak and this is only the case if the information (evidence) they wish to offer arose within specific parameters; that is, as a result of certain research designs and a particular research orientation. Conversely, individuals who wish to critique the evidence-based practice movement may be silenced using terms, such as, rigour, generalisability, control or randomisation.

We can thus see how stratification functions as a component of knowledge development by creating taxonomies, classifying observations and ordering data (Colebrook 2002) according to a governing *epistemè*. It is a method by which an array of disparate and/or similar information can be rendered coherent and thus usable (Colebrook 2002). The questions remain, however: to whom is this information coherent and for whom it is intended? As part of this line of questioning and thinking, Deleuze and Guattari remind us that even the act of describing thoughts, ideas, and objects with language, for example, subjects them to linguistic stratification (Message 2005a). Organising data requires submitting them to a grid, to a pre-existent structure that is based on specific assumptions (or an *epistemè*). In doing so, certain objects – types of knowledge, or forms of knowledge development – are assigned to higher or lower positions in the schema; for example, the assignment of particular study designs and their corresponding findings to the positions of good, better, or best (Holmes et al. 2006a, 2006b). This means that stratification produces a hierarchy, wherein objects are located within space, involving their being ranked in relation to one another (Murray, Holmes and Rail 2008).

Consequently, stratification assumes a political function – most notably because it both produces distinct territories and assigns items to these identifiable areas, with some being elevated to superior positions and others to inferior ones. Often, stratification is quite exclusionary. Some items are accepted; others are outright rejected. When phenomena are clustered, grouped and sorted (even when this is done for ease of comprehension and meaning), this discriminatory process makes prejudiced distinctions resulting in differential treatment and regard of that which is stratified based on its ascribed status (Message 2005b). This can be seen in evidence-based practice where classification is based on a value-laden hierarchy (best and better are judgemental terms), wherein things are not seen as being equal: some are subordinated, others are elevated; some evidence is best, other evidence is sub-optimal. When this happens, when these hierarchies are created and enforced, we are no longer beyond the concept of good and evil (Deleuze 1983); we are in the midst of its construction and implementation because the assignment of good and bad (often euphemised by terms such as optimal and unsatisfactory) can occur only after a particular form of stratification (a given *epistemè*) gains social, scientific and political dominance.

Evidence-Based Practice as a Political Enterprise

To support the claim that evidence-based practice is ultimately a political undertaking, we will now draw on the work of Michel Foucault. While Foucault did not address evidence-based practice specifically, he did argue that scientific discourses, whatever they may be about, conceal power relations through the appropriation of a supposedly absolute and objective truth that not only exists, but also is knowable (Foucault 1997). Science (and for us, evidence-based practice as a component of the health sciences) is a process wherein information is sorted and stratified based on the values and assumptions of those who are: (1) able to establish rules for knowledge and (2) most likely to benefit if knowledge systems remain unchanged.[2] The dogmatic exclusion of alternate modes of thought is a feature of what Foucault calls a regime of truth, a dominant way of seeing the world that seeks recourse in scientific discourse, maintains the effects of hegemony and consolidates the countless institutional structures from which these arise (Holmes, Roy and Perron 2008). The stratification of evidence which underpins evidence-based practice thus precisely generates and maintains a contemporary regime of truth about objectivity.

Foucault states that regimes of truth are based on scientific discourses which, on the one hand, maintain the effects of domination while, on the other hand, strengthen the institutional structures that shape them (Holmes, Murray and Perron 2009). Truth, therefore, is to be understood as a system of ordered procedures (stratifications) for the production, regulation, distribution and circulation of

---

2 It is noteworthy that it is quantitative researchers who proclaim quantitative methods as producing *best* evidence. This forces one to wonder how much of this advocacy is ultimately self-serving.

statements (Foucault 1997). It is that which is accepted within the rigid rules of a dominant *epistemè,* not an absolute, irrefutable, or objective understanding of reality (Foucault 1997).

Moreover, truth is linked in a circular relationship with 'systems of power that produce and sustain it, and to effects of power that induce and extend it' (Foucault 1980: 131). Each society has its own regime of truth (which is maintained and understandable as an *epistemè*). These include: the type of discourse which is accepted; the mechanisms and instances which enable one to distinguish true and false statements; the means by which understandings of the world are sanctioned; the techniques and procedures accorded value in the acquisition of truth; and, the status of those who are charged with saying what counts as true. It is therefore important to understand the constructed nature of truth and power. Consequently, Foucault's genealogical methodology exposes 'the workings of the dominant *epistemè*, bringing to light the implicit strategic apparatuses by which something appears to be true or false, good or bad' (Foucault 1980, 1997, Holmes et al. 2008: 396). We believe that his analysis can be extended to the discourse surrounding the evidence-based practice, helping to reveal 'the complex interactions between organisational, institutional and ethico-political structures' (Holmes et al. 2008: 396).

As part of this intricate system of truth and knowledge production, Foucault (1997) argued that there are multiple discursive regimes, each of which can be traced to particular settings and institutions. Despite these differences, however, each system replicates a similar process: the ideological valorisation of one discourse over others and the ranking of certain types of thinking as better than others (Holmes et al. 2008). As noted above, in the first wave of evidence-based practice this process involved a near total exclusion and rejection of any research methodology or ideation about clinical practice that did not reflect mainstream rules of stratification. Anything that was not complicit and compliant with the dominant *epistemè* was marginalised. While, at times, this process involved an outright rejection of all non-quantitative methodologies and the evidence which arose from them, the actual issue at hand concerned the rules of stratification: how reality could be and was defined; what statements could be uttered regarding good versus bad science and clinical practice; and why certain issues were declared problems while others were not. This process thus led to the establishment of binding norms because such discursive regimes target specific objects of knowledge as surfaces upon which social policies can be inscribed and known (Foucault 1980). These policies result in normalising trends that homogenise thought, discourse and behaviour in the name of a particular ideology (*epistemè*). When resistance against evidence-based practice began to emerge and become widespread across health-related disciplines, however, new strategies were deployed to address this threat. The novel nature of these strategies, which achieve stratification in progressively more subtle and amenable ways, pushed evidence-based practice into its second wave.

The Second Wave of Evidence-Based Practice: The Rise of the Empire

In their book *Empire*, Hardt and Negri (2000) describe the foregoing process of
stratification as an integral component of the contemporary, imperial, political
system. They posit that the contemporary system of global dominance and
governance is based on an increasingly pervasive and exceedingly dense system
of sociopolitical stratification. Items and objects (both animate and inanimate),
which had previously escaped identification and rank, or which were formerly
excluded, have now been incorporated into the empire. Little by little, the social
apparatus defined as the empire, expands, without much resistance primarily due
to a drastic decrease in the emphasis on exclusion.[3] In the health sciences, this
corresponds to the transition from using quantitative/epidemiological methods
only to the proliferation of mixed designs, notwithstanding the nature of research
objectives; that is, the insertion of qualitative techniques into research projects that
have an overarching post-positivistic approach.

For Hardt and Negri, this process of expansion (by means of undifferentiated
inclusion and subsequent stratification) is a political strategy that structures and
regulates life through the inclusion–differentiation–management sequence. To
explain further, the first of these three steps, inclusion, involves the reduction or
elimination of exclusionary practices, such as those evident in the first wave of the
evidence-based practice. For Hardt and Negri, the current imperial model does not
operate on the idea of inside-versus-outside or us-versus-them; rather, its primary
strategy is, first, to include everything and then, second, to deal with that which
has been incorporated. Inclusion is the principal step in this approach because
an acceptance-of-all approach is the method by which the empire guarantees its
expansion. If rapid growth and absolute encapsulation are the goals, then one cannot
afford to exclude. As a result, people may be less likely to resist this expansive
ideology because, at first glance, absolute inclusion (through seduction) is ideal.
Everyone has the ability and right to be an accepted member of the apparatus.
What is often overlooked as part of this process, however, is that after inclusion
occurs, stratification ensues (as in evidence-based practice's first wave). Thus, the
rigid system of evaluating, ranking, and sorting prevails.

This method of stratification, which Hardt and Negri call differentiation, is
the second step in the imperial process. It occurs after inclusion, and is the phase
during which differences that were previously overlooked are clearly identified
and demarcated. At this point, precise differences, right down to the bio-molecular
level if necessary, are identified as signs of uniqueness. They are markings of
exceptional distinction. During this phase, an in-depth examination of all items
within the empire occurs, but not with the goal of exclusion – to exclude at this
point would be antithetical to the first step of absolute inclusion. Consequently,

---

3   This lack of resistance, Hardt and Negri state, arises because the empire's inclusive
façade results in many individuals failing to note that many problems still exist with the
imperial system.

differentiation (stratification) – a process of identifying, listing and ranking the components of the empire – is employed to survey the imperial landscape and to note all that has been incorporated into it. According to Hardt and Negri, however, this does not signal the end of the imperial process.

Instead, immediately after the completion of the inclusion and differentiation processes, management is initiated, during which time strategies to address the array of identified differences are created and implemented, developed and deployed. Again, this is not in an attempt to exclude anyone or anything. Rather, management focuses on the creation of strategies to deal with differences, to enable objects to operate within the overall imperial machine in order to facilitate the continued functioning of the empire. It is during this process of management that each person's or item's unique attributes are addressed to ensure cohesion among them and individual differences are often capitalised on (quite literally; for example, the production of specific products for each of us to consume or use). Precise rules and regulations are then created to guarantee an appropriate continuation of the imperial system. Management thus signals the systematic ordering of that which has been stratified into an organised whole and the coherent utilisation of that which has been thus classified. This is the method by which sorted objects are controlled, mastered and dealt with appropriately.

From our perspective, evidence-based practice in its second wave strongly resembles the imperial process that Hardt and Negri describe. Evidence-based practice not only functions as a component of the contemporary empire, it also employs the three-step sequence: include, differentiate and manage. Evidence-based practice is no longer an exclusionary method of practice, thinking or research – all forms of evidence and most types of knowledge development are now permitted to exist and proliferate within the new evidence-based practice approach: systematic reviews, meta-analysis, randomised controlled, double blind studies, case reports, ideas, editorials, opinions, to name a few, are all recognised as valid. However, these various research approaches are now ranked within the system and some are still relegated to inferior positions within the evidence hierarchy; for example, most qualitative study designs. This ranking system resembles what is sometimes referred to as an evidence pyramid with certain forms, such as those at the beginning of the foregoing list, being designated as superior, better or best forms of evidence. Despite this hierarchy, evidence-based practice displays its new imperial attributes by including all forms of evidence, and later, managing the differences of research design and method by ranking the evidence which arises from these different research approaches; thus, resistance is silenced.

The inclusive nature of evidence-based practice is, therefore, one attribute that makes this method of practice and research highly seductive – and many researchers across the globe have followed this path. Nowhere in evidence-based practice documents does it state that only randomised controlled trials produce the best evidence, or that only the findings of systematic reviews should be used to guide practice. Instead, such research designs are simply elevated to a superior position in certain cases; as noted above, randomised controlled trials are often considered the gold standard for research that examines the efficaciousness of an intervention, while other designs are deemed to be more appropriate in other scenarios. Using the words of Hardt and Negri, it could be suggested that all evidence is accepted (that is, included), then differentiated,and lastly managed based on research design. It is thus possible to understand how evidence-based practiceinduces cooperation and disarms resisting bodies. On the one hand, evidence-based practiceis seen to include all forms of evidence (even though it debases some of them), while on the other hand, evidence-based practice also appears to be a strategy that some claim is, without any doubt, in everyone's (patients', practitioners', funders', *et cetera*) best interests.

We contend, however, that this may not be the case. The political nature of evidence-based practice indicates that it is a mechanism that helps to maintain the current *epistemè*. It is a codified and widely accepted strategy that does not necessarily evaluate which evidence is best for patients. Rather, evidence-based practice discerns which research has been produced according to certain hierarchical rules wherein the evidence that arises from dominant biomedical research designs is elevated to a superior position. Thus, it assesses methodological congruence, not optimal evidence,by evaluating how closely the methods from which the evidence arises correspond with contemporary ideas about research, knowledge and knowledge development. This imperial nature of evidence-based practice reveals that much more is involved than simply evidence and practice; it is a self-perpetuating and ever-expanding system of hierarchy and dominance (Holmes, Roy and Perron 2008) – a process which we believe is ultimately imperialistic in nature.

Resisting the Violence of Stratification: A Note on the War Machines

The political/imperial stratification of research, which we believe constitutes the core of evidence-based practice, should not continue to influence researchers, clinicians and administrators into accepting only one approach to health care practice. Instead, we believe that the situation described above could provide the impetus to challenge the contemporary system of evidence-based stratification and to engage in a form of resistance that Deleuze and Guattari called the war machine. Althusser postulated an epistemological break between ideology and science; however, he considered this to be a critical (evolutionary) process, rather than a sudden revolution (Holmes et al. 2008). Consequently, we argue for the need to question, test and dispute what some might consider the quasi-totalitarian evidence-based practice ideology. In order to ground this refusal to accept one single interpretation and systematisation of reality and health care practice, we return to the political philosophy of Deleuze and Guattari, specifically to their concept of the war machine this time.

For these two authors, the war machine is the metaphorical initiation and performance of resistance. However, this does not signify resistance to one specific cause in an effort to replace it with another. Rather, the war machine represents a rejection of static forms of thinking and behaving, a call to perpetually and continually challenge one's beliefs (which, ironically, may involve rejecting resistance and critique for a period of time, only to resume this process thereafter). This means that the activation of the war machine is motivated by an individual's or group's desire to question and critique all ideologies, rather than to merely replace one rigid belief system with another.[4] Consequently, the war machine cannot be reduced to a specific credo because, as a conviction, it would then become a mechanism of empire – a strategy employed in the imperial system of inclusion, differentiation and management. As a result, the war machine needs to be understood both as a process and a set of tools for questioning, investigating and analysing any system of thought or belief (any stratification, that is). This means that it has no specific principles of its own other than to promote critique and debate; it is simply a focus of resistance to, and critical disruption of, mainstream and dominant ways of being and thinking (Kawash 1998). It is a poststructuralist orientation that focuses on deconstructing dominant *epistemè*.

To further understand Deleuze and Guattari's concept of the war machine, it is important that we first become acquainted with how these authors define the term, concept. Stated simply, to Deleuze and Guattari, 'concepts [such as war machine and/or stratification] are not labels or names that we attach to things; they produce an orientation or a direction for thinking' (Colebrook 2002: 15). Concepts are expansive in that they do not limit, but rather, provide themselves as tools which are ready to be used in opposition to the mainstream, the axiomatic and the dogmatic (Colebrook 2002, Howard 1998). With this clarification, we can understand that stratification is not just a descriptive label that helps to formally define a process, nor is it a simple technical definition; rather, it is a method by which difference can be made finite or infinite as is called for, and as is needed, in the name of resistance.

Thus, while it is the method of choice by which evidence-based practice operates, the concept of stratification could be turned upon itself; that is, it could have its focus inverted to become, in the words of Deleuze and Guattari (1987), a war machine. This might occur if, for example, alternative stratifications were proposed. Different, but equally plausible conceptualisations of research, practice or administration could be constructed and proposed as viable alternatives to evidence-based practice. This does not mean, however, that evidence-based practice should be entirely supplanted by a new strategy because this would simply

---

4   The idea of dissolving all ideologies constitutes little more than a masked ideology in and of itself. It is essentially a dogma that pretends not to be dogmatic. The war machine should not be interpreted in this manner; it is the call to change, even when such a change would promote (for an undetermined period of time) a rejection of change. Indeed, if change were to become the norm, then stagnation would be the act of a war machine.

supplant one ideology with another. Instead, this tactic involves the proliferation of strategies for practice and knowledge development; the creation of an array of options – a toolbox – from which different strategies could be selected based on patient preference, contextual determinants and clinician capabilities. For example, dismantling the evidence-based practice hierarchies, reversing the hierarchies or re-evaluating the entire notion of how information becomes stratified might all be viable options in this process. Similarly, the concept of stratification could be used to reveal the underlying processes that are inherent in evidence-based practice. As has been attempted in this chapter, Deleuze and Guattari's idea could be used to explore the current state of affairs and to critically analyse what this means, both socially and politically, for all domains of health care practice. The outcome, in such cases, however, resembles that of the war machine.

Thus, the war machine is a perpetual and continuous act wherein, at the moment that its goal is achieved (thereby rendering the war machine a captive of the target ideology: the apparatus of capture) it changes form and trajectory and attacks what it used to promote (May 2005). As noted above, the war machine is a process of deconstruction not a system of thought. Consequently, the war machine cannot be reduced to a specific belief system because that would transform it into a mechanism of the prevailing doctrine which it was mobilised to attack. Thus, although the war machine was a proponent of evidence-based practice in the days of Copernicus and Galileo (because it was used to dismantle the absolute authority of the Church), it now fights against evidence-based practice by attempting to sabotage the supremacy and violence of this new form of stratification. In other words, while the idea of basing one's practices on empirical evidence was both novel and threatening to the mainstream systems of thought during the period when the Roman Catholic Church possessed near-absolute authority over knowledge and information in western society, since that time this *epistemè* has become the dominant approach. Consequently, the war machine that Copernicus and Galileo invoked (in the form of practice based on evidence), which ultimately debased the Church, must now be re-engaged and turned upon the current mainstream worldview that threatens to prevent alternative perceptions of the world.

As a response to evidence-based practice, enacting a Deleuzo-Guattarian war machine would involve the active dismantling and dissolution of pyramids of knowledge (the ranking of evidence, that is) and the acknowledgement that when individuals or groups rank evidence, they are often doing so for personal and political gain. In fact, we need to challenge the proponents of evidence-based practice to demonstrate how certain forms of evidence (usually the findings of research methods that they advocate using) produce better clinical outcomes because, while efficacy research is important, the effectiveness of best evidence needs to be considered. The war machine served as an impetus for science centuries ago; now, it is time to ensure that the iconoclastic (war machine) nature of this science does not disappear into a new scientific orthodoxy. Indeed, it is time to deconstruct the constraints of evidence-based practice, not only by examining what sociopolitical constructs are necessary for such an idea to exist but also by exploring alternative ways of being and knowing.

Conclusion

The production of knowledge and its use are forms of social practice that are saturated with politics. In this chapter, we have introduced the politically charged concepts of stratification, the empire and war machines to give form to this resistance. We believe that the very real impact and powerful momentum of the evidence-based practice and best practice guidelines, which pervade the health sciences domain, need to be examined. Rather than being strictly objective or scientific, the evidence-based practice is, above all, a political movement, one that suppresses non-conforming ideas, subjugates some clinicians and exalts others and imposes this method of care to the person in need of care (Holmes et al. 2006a). This power position falls within Foucault's conception of the government of bodies and the standardisation of existence brought on by a specific epistemology: 'This approach bears some resemblance to a regime that does not prohibit one to speak, but forces one to speak in a specific way' (Holmes, Roy and Perron 2008: 49). Accordingly, we challenge the hegemonic influence of evidence-based practice and promote instead a system of multiplicity, change and critique. We do not endorse the abandonment of evidence-based practice (as noted above, we use evidence in our daily research and clinical practice), but its examination and evaluation.

　　Once more, we argue against the hierarchical differentiation of varied research approaches so as to allow diverse methodologies to guide research and ultimately to structure practice. This critique is aimed at an attitude that we feel is largely promoted within the health sciences: that knowledge development can only occur within one paradigm and way of knowing. As some of our colleagues have already argued, health-science discourse must allow multiple perspectives that reflect the actuality of clinical practice (Holmes et al. 2006) because research undertaken within the strict evidence-based logic greatly oversimplifies the complexity of modern health care. Such diminishment may result in the disparagement of alternative (some groundbreaking) research designs permeating all levels of health sciences – from clinical practice to curricula, research funding and scientific journals and databases – all in the name of maintaining the *status quo*. Again, we assert that the evidence-based practice is ideologically driven and, therefore, highly political. Along with Miles, Loughlin and Polychronis (2008: 638), we purport that it is 'entirely possible to conclude that evidence-based practice remains a dogmatic phenomenon, displaying all of the cardinal characteristics of an ideology'. As part of this, we believe that all health care workers (for example, clinicians, researchers, administrators, funders and policy-makers) must consider if certain ways of knowing are, in fact, superior – which means, in short, that what we endorse is a critique of evidence-based practice to ensure that this phenomenon does not cause stagnation or prevent advancement in the health sciences.

References

Cochrane Consumer Network. 2010. *Levels of Evidence.* [Online]. Available at: http://consumers.cochrane.org/levels-evidence [accessed: 30 January 2011].

Colebrook, C. 2002. *Gilles Deleuze.* New York: Routledge.

Davidoff, F., Haynes, B.,Sackett, D. and Smith, R. 1995. Evidence based medicine. *British Medical Journal*, 310, 1085.

Deleuze, G. 1983. *Nietzsche and Philosophy.* New York: The Athlone Press.

Deleuze, G. and Guattari, F. 1987. *A Thousand Plateaus: Capitalism and Schizophrenia.* New York: Continuum Press.

Foucault, M. 1997. *Les mots et les choses.* St-Amand: Tel-Gallimard.

Foucault, M. 1980. *Power/knowledge: Selected Interviews and Other Writings, 1972–1977.* New York: Pantheon.

Hardt, M. and Negri, A. 2000. *Empire.* New York: Harvard University Press.

Holmes, D., Murray, S., and Perron, A. 2009.'Insufficient' but still 'necessary'? EBPM's dangerous leap of faith. *International Journal of Nursing Studies*, 46(5), 749–50.

Holmes, D., Roy, B. and Perron, A. 2008. The use of postcolonialism in the nursing domain: Colonial patronage, conversion and resistance. *Advances in Nursing Science*, 31(1), 42–51.

Holmes, D., Murray, S., Perron, A. and McCabe, J. 2008. Nursing best practice guidelines: Reflecting on the obscene rise of the void. *Journal of Nursing Management*, 16(4), 394–403.

Holmes, D., Murray, S., Perron, A. and Rail, G. 2006a. Deconstructing the evidence-based discourse in health sciences: Truth, power, and fascism. *International Journal of Evidence-Based Health Care*, 4(3), 180–86.

Holmes, D., Murray, S., Perron, A. and Rail, G. 2006b. Towards an understanding of the politics of 'evidence'. *International Journal of Evidence-Based Health Care*, 4(4), 394–5.

Howard, J. 1998. Subjectivity and space: Deleuze and Guattari's BwO in the new world order, in *Deleuze and Guattari: New Mappings in Politics, Philosophy, and Culture*, edited by E. Kaufman and K. Heller. Minneapolis: University of Minnesota Press, 113–26.

Kawash, S. 1998. 415 men: Moving bodies, or, the cinematic politics of deportation, in *Deleuze and Guattari: New Mappings in Politics, Philosophy, and Culture*, edited by E. Kaufman and K. Heller. Minneapolis: University of Minnesota Press, 127–41.

May, T. 2005. *Gilles Deleuze: An Introduction.* New York: Cambridge University Press.

Message, K. 2005a. Stratification, in *The Deleuze Dictionary*, edited by A. Parr. Edinburgh: Columbia University Press, 266–8.

Message, K. 2005b. Territory, in *The Deleuze Dictionary*, edited by A. Parr. Edinburgh: Columbia University Press, 274–6.

Miles, A., Loughlin, M. and Polychronis, A. 2008. Evidence-based healthcare, clinical knowledge and the rise of personalised medicine. *Journal of Evaluation in Clinical Practice*, 14(5), 621–49.

Murray, S., Holmes, D. and Rail, G. 2008. On the constitution and status of 'evidence' in the Health Sciences. *Journal of Research in Nursing*, 13(4), 272–80.

PART II
Evidence in the Clinic

Chapter 4

Communally-Based Evidence in the Emerging Practice of Aorta Implant Surgery

Berit Brattheim, Arild Faxvaag and Aksel Tjora

Introduction

While evidence-based practice is often based on clinical guidelines (systematically developed statements and recommendations to improve the quality of the practice of care and reduce unnecessary variation) new clinical therapies evolve within practice-based clinical communities. Based on our study of the development of aorta implant surgery in Norway we elaborate on the communal aspects influencing the development of clinical therapies. We are especially interested in the complex relationship between guidelines and practice within a context where practice guidelines are regarded as the embodiment of evidence-based medicine (Woolf et al. 1999), protocols and standards are constantly in a state of flux between emerging and established clinical practices (Timmermans and Berg 1997), and guidelines may serve as bases for collective revisions of informal and tacit mindlines (Gabbay and le May 2004).

In the domain of hospital care and surgery, Pope (2002) developed a typology of sources of variation in the selection of patients and the planning and execution of surgical procedures. Pope described three categories of contingency; related to the patient case, the surgeon, or external to these two (for instance access to equipment or other elements in the environment surrounding the work). Pope argued that such contingencies explained some of the tensions between demand for evidence-based practice and the practicalities of surgical work.

This chapter elaborates on the emergence and character of expertise among clinicians providing surgery to patients with *a*bdominal *a*ortic *a*neurysm, or AAA. As of 2010, the conventional surgical technique of accessing and removing the aneurysm through a large incision has been superseded by a less invasive method known as endovascular repair (EVAR) (Chambers et al. 2009). EVAR is the process of accessing the aorta via a small incision in the groin, using a catheter to introduce and attach a prosthesis (an endograft)[1] that covers the aneurysm from within the aorta. Although studies in the field have explored cost effectiveness, patient benefit, appropriateness of care and possible overuse of the EVAR treatment

---

1 The EVAR prosthesis/endograft is a component that might consist of three parts: a main body and two 'legs', sometimes referred to as 'aorta pants'.

(Chambers et al. 2009, Wilt et al. 2006), there has been little focus on the social and material context within which expertise is developed and refined. In this chapter we explore the situatedness of a novel practice, demonstrating how inclusion of patients for treatment creates a state of flux at an early (semi-experimental) stage in the development of this clinical practice while knowledge and expertise are still emerging. We ask the following questions: *What characterises the emergent EVAR evidence? How does the EVAR evidence develop within a particular social, material, technological, and organisational context?* In the following sections, we present the domain of aortic surgery and introduce a theoretical framework for understanding this emergent form of expertise.

Dealing with Aneurysm of the Abdominal Aorta

The prevalence of aneurysms increases with age. Above the age of 60, one in sixteen people will develop an aneurysm with men four times more likely to be affected than women (Singh et al. 2001). The aneurysm is usually discovered through opportunistic screening, typically after a patient has had a radiological examination for some other condition. Once detected, the patient needs to be checked at regular intervals until the size of the aneurysm approaches the threshold for surgery, approximately 5–5.5 cm. The risk of aneurysm rupture is a major concern and contributes to an overall high mortality rate for this condition (Chambers et al. 2009, Singh et al. 2001).

The EVAR procedure is technically demanding. Both patient selection for treatment and the actual insertion of the prosthesis require the coordinated actions of experts from interventional radiology and vascular surgery. AAA patients' suitability for EVAR depends on anatomical features of the aorta, limiting the use of this treatment alternative. However, therapeutic knowledge, the clinicians' personal skills and improvements of prosthesis materials have progressively extended the indication range for this type of surgery (Wilt et al. 2006). Potential advantages of EVAR over open surgery include shorter hospital stay and fewer short and midterm complications (Chambers et al. 2009, Lange et al. 2008).

The Situatedness of Surgical Skills and Knowledge

This chapter builds on Dreyfus' model of skill acquisition (H. Dreyfus 2003, S. Dreyfus 2004) and the knowledge creation model of Nonaka and Takeuchi (Nonaka and Takeuchi 1995, Nonaka, Toyama and Konno 2000). The Dreyfus model provides a source for delineating characteristics of experts' performance, proposing five stages of increasing expertise: novice, advanced beginner, competent, proficient, and expert. The novice typically follows specific rules while at the other end of the spectrum, the expert immediately perceives how to solve a problem with an insightful practical grasp. This model was later extended to include two more stages (H. Dreyfus 2003): the master and the innovator. The master demonstrates a deep involvement in a specific domain, being able to develop his own set of guiding principles. The innovator goes further, striving to expand the margins of the domain. Prior research has demonstrated the relevance of Dreyfus' model in healthcare training. Benner's study of nurse training (2004) has highlighted the importance of situational learning in the skill development that Dreyfus' model describes.

Nonaka and Takeuchi's model complements the Dreyfus' model by explaining how knowledge is created and expanded situationally (Nonaka and Takeuchi 1995, Nonaka, Toyama and Konno 2000). Their model distinguishes between explicit and tacit knowledge. Explicit knowledge can be articulated, documented, and shared. Tacit knowledge, on the other hand, is individual and not easily shared. Their model postulates that knowledge creation requires continuous interactions between tacit and explicit knowledge, proposing four modes of interactivity: socialisation, in which tacit knowledge can be acquired through shared experiences, for example observations and apprenticeship; externalisation, a communicative process in which tacit knowledge is made explicit, for example by collective reflection and concept building; combination, the stepwise processing of sets of explicit knowledge, for example by supplementing existing knowledge with newly created knowledge; finally, internalisation, closely linked to individual learning by doing, is a process through which explicit knowledge is shared and transferred into tacit knowledge. During the study of the EVAR case we found that the communal aspects of expertise, including the transfer of expertise, were especially significant. This observation made Nonaka and Takeuchi's (1995) framework of interaction particularly relevant to our analysis.

As mentioned in the introduction, there is a tension between formal procedures, such as guideline-based care, and informal practice. Therefore, it is relevant to explore how actors within a particular context find evidence for their actions, as well as achieve their objectives. Suchman's (1987) work introduces the relevance of *situatedness* of action, pointing out that an action's course depends on contextual factors, as well as the actors' continual interpretation of the action itself. For actors facing new or challenging situations, rules and procedures tend to guide the course of the specific actions rather than explicitly directing these. Suchman further emphasises the importance of interactive work with face-to-face communication as a means for obtaining consensus in decision-making. Following Suchman, our approach is to explore the relation between knowledge and action by investigating interaction between the EVAR experts as well as between the experts and the context of the action.

Fieldwork

This chapter is based on data from semi-structured interviews with expert clinicians from one university hospital and two local hospitals that all sit within the jurisdiction of one of Norway's four regional health enterprises. We conducted 12 semi-structured interviews with clinicians. These included three interventional radiologists and three vascular surgeons from the university hospital, all being members of the multidisciplinary EVAR team. From the county hospital we interviewed two vascular surgeons and four radiologists. Since we were concerned with the clinicians' experiences with and *accounts* (Dingwall 1997) of establishing the practice of EVAR therapy, we focus mainly on the empirical material collected at the university hospital to illustrate the particular issues in question. The interview guide was adjusted after the observation study (Brattheim, Seim and Faxvaag 2008) and focused on:

1. AAA care trajectory and the clinical decision-making
2. knowledge creation and dissemination of the EVAR experiences, and
3. future prospects of the EVAR method.

Each interview lasted 45–60 minutes and was audio-recorded for subsequent transcription.

The analysis has been inspired by a grounded theory approach (Strauss and Corbin 1998) and followed an inductive strategy (Creswell 1998). The first step involved generating initial thematic codes. The second step, guided by the theoretical frameworks (H. Dreyfus 2003, S. Dreyfus 2004, Nonaka and Takeuchi 1995, Nonaka, Toyama and Konno 2000), involved grouping these codes into categories and subcategories. Drawing on Suchman's framework (1987), we mapped out three main categories of contextual factors that were relevant for decision-making, which we have identified as interrelated EVAR expertise traits; the collective, the interpersonal, and the technical.

The Collective Trait

Although clinical practice guidelines are widely promoted as a means to standardize practice, the surgeons at the university hospital took somewhat different approaches. Surgeons questioned the need for formal guidelines, claiming that one should avoid making the simple more complicated. Instead, they emphasised the value of collective, informal guiding principles that emerged from years of practice. They described how this collective expertise developed through participation in regular regional and national conferences that supported the sharing of EVAR experience and results at a national level. In-house, the actors worked out basic attitudes through informal and formal discussion, creating an informal common ground, or consensus, to guide practice:

To build guidelines from an analysis of our clinical practice would be a fairly complicated effort. An uncomplicated issue becomes more complicated when rules are written on a piece of paper. (University hospital, surgeon 1)

If you have met one vascular surgeon, you have met them all ... It is a very small and close community, so guidelines are typically developed internally in the group ... Within the same community, we may find slightly differing views. But, by large, the opinions of Norwegian surgeons do not differ much. There might however be 'camps' that are more or less in favour of the technique. In general, the basic attitudes toward whom to treat or not treat tend to be very much in line. (University hospital, surgeon 2)

The surgeons stressed the need to tailor the care to the individual patient's needs. Moreover, the initial assessment of the surgical intervention threshold included a trade-off between multiple factors including, but not limited to, aneurysm size and growth rate, anatomy of the aorta, co-morbidities, patient preferences and the patient's overall life expectancy.

The aneurysm size acted as a guiding factor, but the guideline diameter for surgery, which had been established by the surgeons collectively, was not applied strictly. Instead, the surgeons referred to decision-making as a process of risk assessment, guided by a 'rule of thumb':

As long as the diameter of the aneurysm is smaller than 5 cm, the surgery itself is riskier than not treating the disease – this is the rule of thumb ... However, there is room for individual assessment. Given a patient, age 55 and with serious co-morbidities ... this favours a stentgraft [an EVAR]. If the patient suffers from a heart disease, lung disease or another illness that adds to the risks of open surgery we would argue against open surgery. The decisions must be adapted to the individual patient. (University hospital, surgeon 3)

We make a risk assessment in which we compare the risk of living with the aneurysm with that of surgery. And, in the end, [the outcome of the risk assessment] is crucial to the decision about whether or not to perform surgery. (University hospital, surgeon 1)

Even if the surgeons were responsible for the initial identification of eligible EVAR candidates, the radiologists took an active part in decision-making. The decision on patients' suitability for EVAR took place as a collaborative process during the regular morning conference that involved the teams of interventional radiologists and vascular surgeons. CT scans as well as information about the patient's clinical status provided important bases for decision-making.

Deciding whether or not to select a patient might incorporate a second iteration of EVAR assessment, for instance, when dealing with a high-risk patient. Experts reported that, in many situations, actors sought to extend the 'rule of thumb' for anatomic suitability for EVAR as this could benefit high-risk patients found to be unfit for open surgery. Some of the experts mentioned that the high risk itself reduced life expectancy, independent of the aneurysm parameters. In other words, compared with a healthier patient, the uncertainty about the long-term effect of EVAR was of less concern:

> When the patient is in good health [except for the aneurysm], the anatomical features must be close to perfect before we perform an EVAR. However, in the case of a seriously ill patient at the threshold of being unfit for open surgery or even found to be completely unfit for the open repair alternative, we might extend the margins beyond the recommended anatomical inclusion criteria for EVAR. This makes sense as the life expectancy for such a patient is relatively poor – independent of the aneurysm. As an AAA patient with a severe heart disease is only expected to live a few years, the durability of the EVAR is not so much a cause for concern as in the situation of an otherwise healthy patient. (University hospital, radiologist 3)

Furthermore, the clinicians indicated that high-risk patients found unfit for any major surgery, should terminate the aneurysm surveillance program. However, some patients, aware of the severity of the condition, opted to remain in the program. In some cases, the surgeons could revise their decisions not to operate:

> If neither open surgery nor EVAR can be recommended, the surveillance program should be terminated. But some patients are very uncomfortable with this decision; I believe they might feel abandoned. Several patients therefore want to remain in the program. In the case of a rapidly progressing aneurysm – and even if we initially decided not to operate on the aneurysm – we might reconsider and try to stretch the limits even further. (University hospital, radiologist 3)

> Through practical experience, I have become less categorical. If the [X-ray] report states that 'the patient is anatomically suited', the patient's aneurysm is actually suited for a stent graft. Otherwise, we use phrases like 'not optimal' or 'stentgrafting is possible' ... And yes, we also use such phrases as 'stentgrafting is impossible ...'. If we report that stentgrafting is impossible, there is no way that the patient can get an EVAR. Sometimes, we intentionally make ambiguous descriptions. (University hospital, radiologist 3)

The practice of reversing decisions whether or not to operate even influenced how the radiologist assessed the CT images. In some cases, the radiologist was deliberately vague in the phrasing of the assessment of suitability in order to consider a future reassessment of EVAR.

The experts advocated a master-apprentice approach as an important instrument for developing skills, emphasising the importance of hands-on training performed in a day-to-day situation. However, the formal surgical training program did not include any specific EVAR requirements. Moreover, not every surgeon appeared to be a candidate for EVAR training. Within the interventionist team, the EVAR practitioners seemed to practice an informal, but still systematic, training program. In principle, the radiologists would regard most EVAR procedures as training events:

> It is not required that every vascular surgeon should be able to perform the EVAR procedure. ... Earlier, a vascular surgeon had to demonstrate a strong interest before he was allowed to participate. Nowadays, when we have fewer experts, getting access to the field is perhaps slightly easier than before ... but not all who wish to perform EVAR gets to. (University hospital, surgeon 2)

> There is no formal training plan for the performance of EVAR. You build your experience gradually. (University hospital, radiologist 2)

The current work practice appeared to encourage collective learning and skill acquisition. However, the apprenticeship program that the clinicians mentioned took place mainly as an internal activity within each professional group.

The Interpersonal Trait

In Norway, the novel EVAR treatment was introduced in 1995. Two enthusiastic experts – a vascular surgeon and an interventional radiologist – became the driving forces of its further development. To exemplify, the initial prostheses consisted of customised 'home-made' devices prepared in close collaboration between the two experts. Gradually, this partnership expanded to encompass a larger interdisciplinary community, with teams consisting of five or six experts in vascular surgery and interventional radiology, respectively. The clinicians outlined how relationship and interpersonal interactions played a major role in the EVAR practice, for instance in repeated negotiations of EVAR assessments for high-risk patients:

> When we prepare for the interdisciplinary meeting, we have made up our minds about the patient's [anatomical] suitability for EVAR. And, some [patients] have an aorta that is perfectly suited, and then we state this. Today, one of my patients was this way; the aorta was wonderful! We say that EVAR is possible, also that [the vascular surgeons] have to talk with the patient [to get consent] ... Then we have some [patients], to whom we say: 'EVAR is possible, but he is not well-suited', we have many of these [patients] actually; a majority of the patients belong to this category. Then the vascular surgeons would argue: 'But ... this patient is very ill. He suffers from angina or has undergone heart surgery, he even suffers from chronic pulmonary disease; we consider open surgery to be too risky.' Then we will answer: 'Well – yes – in that situation we believe

we can make it', and given that answer, we have decided to perform the EVAR
procedure. But, some patients are completely unsuited for EVAR, i.e. when their
aorta lacks specific features like the upper [aortic] neck, or if the arteries in the
groin are too calcified, we say that EVAR is impossible. (University hospital,
radiologist 3)

Although this discussion was essential to ensure a collective, consensus-based
decision on patient suitability for EVAR, the face-to-face discussion revealed that
the individual experts preferred explaining and justifying personal views in a rather
informal manner. As an example, the radiologists immediately recognised 'the
right patient with the right anatomy'. The radiologist did not go into details, but
instead concentrated on some nuances of phrasing, like 'perfect' and 'wonderful',
reflecting an 'intuitive grasp of the situation' (H. Dreyfus 2003). Further, the
presence of multiple interactions accounted for other types of informal information
exchange between individual clinicians. For instance, the empirical data reflect
episodes in which the surgeon contacted a colleague to obtain their view on a
specific patient's surgical condition. Likewise, having obtained a patient's consent
on EVAR, the surgeon passed on the information to one of the radiologists – either
by phone or face-to-face – informing the radiologist to proceed with further EVAR
related tasks.

As for the national vascular surgery environment, our surgeons described this
to be rather small. They suggested that personal knowledge and relationships
played an important role in their professional development and that informal
discussions supported the sharing of 'a common ground':

> We are a small community, with a lot of informal discussions and dialogues. We
> have many informal meetings … we know each other well, but we are also well
> aware of discussions elsewhere. And we bring these back home and continue to
> discuss the topics with our colleagues here at the hospital. (University hospital,
> surgeon 2)

The Technical Trait

Technical improvements of the EVAR prosthesis facilitated the progress of EVAR,
thereby leading to a specialisation of tasks between the two expert teams. The
radiologists – being the experts in introducing the prosthesis through the veins –
took responsibility for tasks related to the prosthesis. Moreover, the radiologists
reported that the implementation of the EVAR procedure involved significant
challenges, in particular when anatomy or pathology rendered difficulties. For
these actors, the EVAR procedure was not merely an act of treatment as it required
ongoing problem-solving. The continuous accumulation of experiences was
essential for solving future specific problems such as when deciding whether a
patient was anatomically suited for EVAR:

When the interdisciplinary meeting has concluded that [EVAR] should be performed, we take note of the name and [national identification] number of the patient. Thereafter, we continue with requesting the graft. We have to 'post-process' the CT images to obtain the right measurements of the aorta and the prosthesis. (University hospital, radiologist 2)

You need detailed knowledge about the various components [of the prosthesis] – you will have to read the product specifications [brochures]. However, merely reading the brochures does not suffice. You must assess the rigidity and the degree of resistance in the blood vessel. If the vessel is not too calcified, it still might be possible to position the guide wire. Remember, the blood vessel might be very curvy. Again, practical experience is required to be able to assess whether or not you think the guide wire can be positioned during a potential endovascular intervention. You have to be competent in handling the guide wire before you go on with the selection of prosthesis. A wide-range diffusion of this specific knowledge will not do any good. (University hospital, radiologist 2)

Hence, expertise is not only bodily embedded and an art, but also technically mediated: hands-on skills with the particular stentgraft material that is adjusted for the size of each particular patient's aorta are prerequisites for successful treatment. Still, some skills become routine, for example the management of prosthesis, the skill training for selecting components and keeping basic prosthesis parts in stock for emergency cases:

Usually, we keep a stock of five to six main [prosthesis] bodies with different diameters. These are not tailored to any specific patient. However, the length of the [prosthesis] is selected to fit the majority of the patients. ... If we have a patient with an acute aneurysm rupture, we might apply the prosthesis set, even if it is dedicated to another patient. We would just order another set. (University hospital, radiologist 3)

The clinician's ability to master the skills within the advanced EVAR method did not depend on which hospital had provided the intervention skill training. As one of the radiologists stated, any differences in practice were related to the individual expert's specific beliefs and preferences with respect to how to 'get from A to B':

It depends on the beliefs of the individual clinician. Some emphasise that the upper neck of the aorta, which should be employed to the prosthesis' main body, does not slide. Others pay more attention to avoid 'the pants from slipping down' [i.e., that the leg devices are not properly employed to the body device]. Like all other products, there seem to be some prostheses that prove to be good, and others that do not. Good products tend to stay in the market. Otherwise, they disappear quite quickly – like the old [name] prosthesis. (University hospital, radiologist 2)

Throughout the interviews, radiologists emphasised the fact that actors undertaking EVAR training had to demonstrate a certain level of skill before being allowed to perform independently. To fulfil the basic criteria, the individual expert should be able to recognise and respond appropriately to unexpected events.

Discussion: The Communal Aspects of Clinical Evidence

This study has explored the situatedness of emerging surgical evidence, demonstrating that the EVAR experts' practice is more influenced by the situation at hand than by formal criteria. Our study highlights that the development of EVAR depended on three main contextual factors: patient characteristics, technical artefacts, and a joint decision approach. Among these, the first one, patient characteristics, included aneurysm parameters, various types of co-morbidities, age, gender, and patient preferences. The second contextual factor, technical artefacts included continuous improvements of prosthesis material as well as advances in radiological imaging technology. The third contextual factor, the joint decision approach, included the crossing of technical artefacts and patient characteristics. Our findings also demonstrate how a minority of experts pushed the EVAR procedure even further, and in this role accounted for a set of expertise traits developing within these contexts: the collective, the interpersonal, and the technical. Although collective internalised guiding principles supported patterns of work in the absence of formalised guidelines, the interpersonal trait reflected how the EVAR experts depended on multiple interactions when dealing with the important patient selection for EVAR. In addition, the technical trait demonstrated the importance of the individual clinician's interventional skills combined with the capability to map radiological image interpretations on to the tailoring of prostheses and patient anatomy. Based on these findings, we argue that the notion of a community of guidance is useful for illustrating the continuity of an emerging surgical therapy. We suggest that surgical evidence in new therapies are secured without formalised institutions, training, or guidelines, and that evidence must be thought of as communal.

The study reported on here reinforces previous findings around the nature of evidence-based medicine (EBM) and use of clinical practice guidelines (Gabbay and le May 2004, Pope 2002). Thus, we suggest that within a technology-intensive environment the EVAR experts take their set of guiding principles even further, often challenging the margins of the surgical domain. To illustrate, in contrast to Pope's (2002) work on the typology of contingencies, our findings demonstrate how external contingency becomes highly prominent in surgical practice: First, the EVAR treatment itself is contingent on (a) the need for customised prosthesis to fit the individual patient's anatomy and (b) the continual technical development of the prosthesis. Second, the iterative (in)formal interaction between radiologists and surgeons enables actors to stretch the margins when reassessing the trade-off between the uncertain durability of the prosthesis itself and the risk of surgical treatment. Third, patient preferences influence decisions; for the high-risk patient, the EVAR technique might represent another chance of being cured. Finally, the adoption of the EVAR method is organisationally embedded. As pointed out by Broom, Adams and Tovey (2009), organisational structures create variation in the impact of evidence in clinical practice. Moreover, at the university hospital, in-house experts are capable of initiating EVAR therapy and push innovation further. The Norwegian regulation of the healthcare system supports this, by legitimising the introduction of medical advances at a university hospital before transferring knowledge, technologies, and methods to local hospitals.

Our analysis suggests the importance of community for the continued development of an evolving surgical therapy. Of major relevance for this perspective are Lave and Wenger's (1991) emphasis on how apprenticeship promotes learning through participation in a shared practice. We have illustrated that within the EVAR team, the collective expertise trait relied on an informal apprenticeship program that allowed trainees to acquire EVAR skills. Furthermore, we observed how EVAR experts establish a shared context in which each expert articulates forms of tacit knowledge through the use of metaphors and figurative phrases. In this way, these actors promoted mutual understanding and acceptance as a basis for the subsequent course of action (Nonaka and Takeuchi 1995). Wenger's work on community of practice (1998) follows a similar approach, suggesting that multiple interactions are prerequisites for making sense of explicit knowledge and creating a shared understanding. The interpersonal expertise trait, as suggested in this study, also reflects the presence of relationships and strong social ties; in other words, how the implicit (re)negotiation of the limits of EVAR therapy is situated (Suchman 1987) in any (in)formal encounter between clinicians. Moreover, social ties become essential for sharing in-depth expertise as well as pushing innovative processes (Hakkarainen 2004, Nonaka, Toyama and Konno 2000). The community of guidance is based on such social ties among clinicians and forms a basis for shared understanding, socialisation/training through participation and reliable clinical practice. An important observation is that the community of guidance supports clinicians in their practical patient assessment, taking into account that inclusion criteria for EVAR therapy are complex and in flux.

On the basis of our analysis, we put forward that in order to understand the phenomenon of emerging clinical evidence, one must look at various traits of expertise, how these are formed on a communal basis, as well as the contextual factors of patient characteristics, technical artefacts, and decision-making approaches. Context-dependent knowledge is often very difficult to transfer (Dopson et al. 2003, Hakkarainen 2004, Nonaka, Toyama and Konno 2000, Wenger 1998). We argue that the diffusion of EVAR requires close integration and continued interaction between the dual types of expertise. As for the technical expertise trait, the clinicians at local hospitals did not benefit from the technical embodied knowledge of their EVAR colleagues. Recent studies (Baker, Atlas and Afendulis 2008, Levy 2008) have pointed out the importance of a technological environment on clinical practice performance, but do also question technological advances that produce a benefit for only a very few patients, contributing to limited population-level outcome. This critique may also be applied to EVAR therapy. To exemplify, experts in the UK and Italy question patients' access to EVAR due to the need for standardized training programs, national guidelines, and improved financial regulation to run the clinical practice (Cao et al. 2007, Harris 2007). Hence, there is no standard process for the adoption of surgical innovations. Since surgical innovations not only improve healthcare outcomes but also pose economic, ethical, and priority challenges in healthcare provision, the situatedness of surgical innovation should be a topic of political concern.

Concerning the technical expertise, our findings reflect a strong focus on the further development of prostheses (Wilt et al. 2006). In fact, some high-risk patients who are turned down for open surgery continued to be monitored in anticipation of future improvement of the EVAR technology. The complex nature of EVAR practice changed the radiologist's role from diagnostic, to technological, to therapeutic. Hence, the interventional radiologist became a vital member of the AAA care team and in this way affected the professional power structures. Comparable international studies of the EVAR practice have shown that it is the vascular surgeon that most predominantly undertakes EVAR procedures (Danjoux et al. 2007, Espinosa 2007). One reason for variations across countries is the conflicting views within medical disciplines regarding ownership of the EVAR innovation. Another is the surgeons' development of new skill sets in intervention that render the radiologists superfluous when performing EVAR procedures. In Norway, however, radiologists and surgeons have collaborated very closely since the beginning of EVAR and the interdependence between these disciplines is an integral part of the community of guidance. Consequently, ownership of the EVAR innovation itself, including materials, processes, techniques, and history, is also integrated in the community, but with national variations on the reach of the communal aspect of evidence. While the community of practice (Lave and Wenger 1991) focuses on human actors, the community of guidance includes human actors, their interdependencies and relations, as well as relevant tasks, tools and materials. It is not only individual skills and collaboration that guide the practice and limits of EVAR therapy, but also institutional arrangements (or lack thereof), prosthesis materials, and patient characteristics. Hence, the community of guidance is situated within these social and material constraints and potentialities. Although there is always risk involved in therapy at an experimental stage, this risk is reduced through communal consensus on matters such as when to stretch (and not to stretch) inclusion criteria for EVAR therapy.

One challenge that remains is that the number of suitable patients may be low. In this case, low patient volume, cost concerns, too few technical improvements and a lack of driving forces appear to challenge further progress of EVAR. At the macro level the contextual influence seems to be weaker. The evolving EVAR knowledge does not easily find its way across organisational borders. Consequently, lack of information and knowledge at the local level has made it more difficult for clinicians at local hospitals to identify eligible EVAR candidates. The identification of such problems also supports the community of guidance concept. Although materials, methods, and inclusion criteria are dynamic within the community, the community itself, and its borders, is fairly static. Guidelines for EVAR therapy diffuse organically from within the specialist community rather than (as formal requirements) from health authorities. Hence, in university hospitals, *communities of guidance* evolve, with an implicit blessing from national regulating authorities. As a result, clinicians who wish to solve challenging problems are allowed to push innovation. Despite the emphasis on RCTs and EBM in medical research and health service delivery, our study demonstrates that socially situated enthusiasm, well fertilised within a community of guidance, pushes methods and technologies forward in surgical practice. While the broad scale application of new clinical therapies rests upon solid formal evidence, the case of EVAR therapy demonstrates that evidence as communal may secure medical treatment in the often very long period of technological-surgical development.

Acknowledgments

We wish to thank the surgeons and radiologists from the three case hospitals who were willing to participate in the study. The study was approved by the Regional Committee for Medical Research Ethics and the Norwegian Social Science Data Services (NSD). The physicians in charge granted access to the field. We obtained signed informed consent from all participants. We would also like to thank Andreas Landmark for technical help with the manuscript. Parts of this chapter were originally published by Sage in the journal *Health* (London) December 2010 (doi: 1363459310376300) in a paper titled 'Getting the aorta pants in place: A community of guidance in the evolving practice of vascular implant surgery'. Permission to reprint licence number: 2665761023361.

References

Baker, L.C., Atlas, S.W. and Afendulis, C.C. 2008. Expanded use of imaging technology and the challenge of measuring value. *Health Affairs*, 27(6), 1467–78.

Brattheim, B., Seim, A.R. and Faxvaag, A. 2008. Clinical processes in an innovative vascular surgeon community: Implications for workflow modeling. *Studies in Health Technology and Informatics*, 136, 371–6.

Broom, A., Adams, J. and Tovey, P. 2009. Evidence-based healthcare in practice: A study of clinician resistance, professional de-skilling, and inter-speciality differentiation in oncology. *Social Science and Medicine*, 68 (1), 192–200.

Cao, P., De Rango, P., Parlani, G. and Verzini, F. 2007. *EVAR in Italy: National Directives Needed for EVAR in Italy.* [Online: Endovascular Today]. Available at: http://www.bmctoday.net/evtoday/ [accessed: 23 March 2010].

Chambers, D., Epstein, D., Walker, S., Fayter, D., Paton, F., Wright, K., Michaels, J., Thomas, S., Sculpher, M. and Woolacott, N. 2009. Endovascular stents for abdominal aortic aneurysms: A systematic review and economic model. *Health Technology Assessment*, 13, 48.

Creswell, J.W. 1998. *Qualitative Inquiry and Research Design: Choosing Among Five Traditions.* London: Sage Publications.

Danjoux, N.M., Martin, D.K., Lehoux, P.N., Harnish, J.L., Shaul, R.Z., Bernstein, M. and Urbach, D.R. 2007. Adoption of an innovation to repair aortic aneurysms at a canadian hospital: A qualitative case study and evaluation. *BMC Health Services Research*, 7, 182.

Dingwall, R. 1997. Accounts, interviews and observations, in *Context and Method in Qualitative Research*, edited by G. Miller and R. Dingwall. London: Sage Publication.

Dopson, S., Locock, L., Gabbay, J., Ferlie, E. and Fitzgerald, L. 2003. Evidence-based medicine and the implementation gap. *Health*, 7(3), 311–30.

Dreyfus, H.L. 2003. *From Novice to Expert.* Lecture given at Norwegian School of Sport Science, DVD. Oslo: Norwegian School of Sport Sciences.

Dreyfus, S.E. 2004. The five-stage model of adult skill acquisition. *Bulletin of Science Technology Society*, 24(3), 177–81.

Espinosa, G. 2007. *An Increasing EVAR Population.* [Online: Endovascular Today]. Available at: http://www.bmctoday.net/evtoday/ [accessed: 23 March 2010].

Gabbay, J. and le May, A. 2004. Evidence-based guidelines or collectively constructed 'mindlines?' ethnographic study of knowledge management in primary care. *British Medical Journal*, 329(7473), 1013.

Hakkarainen, K. 2004. *Communities of Networked Expertise: Professional and Educational Perspectives.* Amsterdam: Elsevier.

Harris, P. 2007. *EVAR in the United Kingdom: A Management Model in Need of Revision.* [Online: Endovascular Today]. Available at: http://www.bmctoday.net/evtoday/ [accessed: 23 March 2010].

Knoblauch, H. 2005. Focused ethnography. *Forum: Qualitative Social Research*, 6(3), article no 44. Available at: http://www.qualitative-research.net/index.php/fqs/article/view/20/44 [accessed: 15 March 2011].

Lange, C., Aasland, J.K., Ødegård, A. and Myhre, H. 2008. The durability of EVAR – what are the evidence and implications on follow-up? *Scandinavian Journal of Surgery*, 97(2), 205–12.

Lave, J. and Wenger, E. 1991. *Situated Learning: Legitimate Peripheral Participation.* Cambridge: Cambridge University Press.

Levy, P. 2008. Adapting process-improvement techniques in an academic medical center. *The Bridge*, 38(1), 6–9.

Nonaka, I. and Takeuchi, H. 1995. *The Knowledge-Creating Company: How Japanese Companies Create the Dynamics of Innovation.* New York: Oxford University Press.

Nonaka, I., Toyama, R. and Konno, N. 2000. SECI, Ba and leadership: A unified model of dynamic knowledge creation. *Long Range Planning*, 33(1), 5–34.

Pope, C. 2002. Contingency in everyday surgical work. *Sociology of Health and Illness*, 24(4), 369–84.

Singh, K., Bonaa, K.H., Jacobsen, B.K., Bjork, L. and Solberg, S. 2001. Prevalence of and risk factors for abdominal aortic aneurysms in a population-based study: The Tromso Study. *American Journal of Epidemiology*, 154(3), 236–44.

Strauss, A.L. and Corbin, J.M. 1998. *Basics of Qualitative Research: Techniques and Procedures for Developing Grounded Theory.* Newbury Park: Sage Publications Inc.

Suchman, L.A. 1987. *Plans and Situated Actions: The Problem of Human-Machine Communication.* Cambridge: Cambridge University Press.

Timmermans, S. and Berg, M. 1997. Standardization in action: Achieving local universality through medical protocols. *Social Studies of Science*, 27(2), 273–305.

Wenger, E. 1998. *Communities of Practice: Learning, Meaning, and Identity.* Cambridge: Cambridge University Press.

Wilt, T., Lederle, F., Macdonald, R., Jonk, Y., Rector, T. and Kane, R. 2006. *Comparison of Endovascular and Open Surgical Repairs for Abdominal Aortic Aneurysm.* Evidence Report/Technology Assessment, no 144. Rockville: Agency for Healthcare Research and Quality.

Woolf, S., Grol, R., Hutchinson, A., Eccles, M. and Grimshaw, J. 1999. Clinical guidelines: Potential benefits, limitations, and harms of clinical guidelines. *British Medical Journal*, 318, 527–30.

Chapter 5

Embodied, Embedded and Encoded Knowledge in Practice: The Role of Clinical Interpretation in Neurorehabilitation

Rob Flynn, Joanne Greenhalgh, Andrew Long and Sarah Tyson

Introduction

Throughout western healthcare systems, there has been a proliferation in the guidelines and protocols that regulate clinical decision-making. Increasingly, clinicians have been required to adhere to codified and explicit procedures and to measure their performance against specific health outcome indicators. This chapter shows how standardised health outcome measures for neurorehabilitation patients are used within a multi-disciplinary team, and how tacit knowledge is intrinsic to this process. Professionals' interpretations of the meanings of certain outcome measurements, such as the Barthel Index and other measurements of patients' functional abilities, are dependent upon other kinds of taken-for-granted knowledge. Clinicians adjust individual patients' scores – and ostensible changes in them – in the light of their clinical judgement and contextual circumstances. Thus, encoded knowledge is explicated, supplemented and sometimes challenged by embedded and tacit knowledge. This chapter outlines the nature and importance of tacit knowledge; it summarises the linkage between evidence-based medicine and health outcome measures and presents qualitative case-study evidence about the uses of outcome measurement in neurorehabilitation. The conclusions reiterate the inevitability of tacit knowledge and the limitations this places on the pursuit of standardisation.

The Nature and Importance of Tacit Knowledge

Many commentators have acknowledged that in almost all aspects of social life, but especially in the context of professional expertise, an important distinction can be made between formal and tacit knowledge. Polanyi (1958), most importantly, discussed scientific knowledge and the role of experimentation. In describing the art of knowing, Polanyi noted that there are certain pre-suppositions used as an interpretive framework. He argued that we dwell in these pre-suppositions much as we do in our own bodies, but they are 'essentially inarticulable' (Polanyi 1958:

60), so, much of this knowledge is 'unspecifiable' (Polanyi 1958: 62). He referred to the skills and connoisseurship necessary to undertake many apparently simple tasks – including cycling, swimming and the use of tools – and how difficult it is for the practitioner to explain what or how that task is accomplished. In relation to science, Polanyi suggested that theoretical and formal knowledge always co-existed alongside what he termed personal knowledge, and that in science we live in personal knowledge that consists of a 'subsidiary awareness of particulars' and 'enables the performance of a skilful achievement' (Polanyi 1958: 64). Polanyi furthered this argument in *The Tacit Dimension* (1983) claiming that it is 'impossible to account for the nature and justification of knowledge by a series of strictly explicit operations' (Polanyi 1983: x) and remarking 'we can know much more than we can tell' (Polanyi 1983: 4). He emphasised the distinction between two types of knowing – knowing *what* and knowing *how* – and insisted that 'neither is ever present without the other' (Polanyi 1983: 4). The procedure of knowing and acting includes both theoretical and practical knowledge. For Polanyi, tacit knowledge 'dwells in our awareness of particulars while bearing upon an entity which the particulars constitute' (Polanyi 1983: 61). Consequently, the search for an impersonal and objective form of abstract knowledge was fruitless. Moreover, 'the process of formalizing all knowledge to the exclusion of any tacit knowledge is self-defeating' (Polanyi 1983: 20). He was also critical of the natural and physical sciences for appearing to subscribe to the view that science was simply a collection of observable facts. In challenging this view as a fallacy, he uses the example of diagnosing a disease: 'facts' necessarily require interpretation, and judgements are not solely based on the available facts – other forms of knowledge, and especially tacit knowledge, are also used.

Many other writers have developed and applied similar insights. Bittner (1974), for example, highlighted the crucial importance of tacit knowledge in organisations. For organisations to work – or more precisely for people to accomplish organisation – tacit assumptions and taken-for-granted knowledge are used constantly. As Bittner noted, within organisations there is: 'a rich and ambiguous body of background information that normally competent members of society take for granted as commonly known'. Normally this information provides:

> the tacit foundation for all that is explicitly known and *provides the matrix for all deliberate considerations without itself being deliberately considered* ... the information enters into that commonplace and practical orientation to reality which members regard as 'natural'. (Bittner 1974: 73 [our emphasis])

Bittner emphasises the importance of unexplicated understandings in organisational work, and also points out that they are essential in the craft and skill necessary to manoeuvre within formal rules.

This dynamic relationship with rules was also explored by Collins (1993) in his account of the structures of knowledge. Collins distinguished between four types of knowledge:

1. symbol-type knowledge: for example, that which can be transferred onto floppy discs
2. embodied knowledge: for example, the co-ordination of thought and movement used in sport and other activities (including medicine and physiotherapy)
3. embrained knowledge: refers to cognitive knowledge and abilities influenced by the physical properties of the brain
4. encultured knowledge: for example, languages.

Collins argued that there are skills that cannot be performed expertly simply by following sets of explicit rules. Such skills have to be learned and then transferred through interpersonal contacts and socialisation within a group. Tacit knowledge is part of this and may be acquired through apprenticeship. Moreover, Collins also points out that there is a 'fundamental division' (Collins 1993: 116) between such tacit knowledge and formal (or encoded) knowledge.

Nonaka (1994) built upon Polanyi's account of tacit knowledge to explain the processes through which organisational knowledge is created. He distinguished tacit knowledge from explicit knowledge, where explicit knowledge consists of codified knowledge which is transmittable into formal, systematic, language. Within organisations, there is an interaction between different forms of knowledge in practice. In ideal-type form, Nonaka identified four types of knowledge conversion within an organisation:

1. from tacit knowledge to other forms of tacit knowledge, such as experienced in 'on-the-job' training or apprenticeships
2. from explicit knowledge to other types of explicit knowledge, such as the information exchanged in computerised databases
3. from tacit knowledge to explicit knowledge such as having to explain the use of standard operating procedures to other organisation members or external audiences
4. from explicit knowledge to tacit knowledge, such as occurs in the process of learning and internalising guidelines.

Tacit knowledge is connected with personal experience and is difficult to formalise or even communicate; it often comprises 'know-how', derives from action and is linked with specific contexts. While it is usually conceived of as an individual or personal concept, tacit knowledge emerges out of shared experience in an organisational setting. Importantly, Nonaka saw organisational learning as benefiting from a continuous interaction between tacit and explicit knowledge. Indeed Nonaka and van Krogh (2009) emphasise that tacit and explicit knowledge occupy a *continuum*. Explicit knowledge has a universal character, whereas tacit knowledge 'is rooted in actions, procedures, routines, commitment, ideals, values and emotions' (Nonaka and van Krogh 2009: 636).

In applying these ideas to organisational cultures, Blackler (1995) extended Nonaka's concepts and also developed Collins' (1993) model of knowledge types, to explain the relationship between knowledge workers or experts, innovation and market competition. He proposed a typology that identified four types of knowledge and four types of organisation that created various admixtures of knowledge-types. Blackler's typology distinguished:

1. embrained knowledge which depends upon conceptual skills and cognitive abilities and is expressed in abstract knowledge (knowledge about or knowledge what)
2. embodied knowledge arises in, and out of, action, and is acquired by doing or problem-solving in specific contexts (knowledge how)
3. embedded knowledge based upon organisational routines
4. encoded knowledge that consists of information conveyed by signs, symbols, books, manuals, codes of practice.

Blackler (1995) argued that expert-dependent organisations (professional bureaucracies such as hospitals) depend upon embodied knowledge. Routinised organisations depend heavily upon embedded knowledge (through rules and procedures). Entrepreneurial or problem-solving organisations depend largely on embrained knowledge. Communication-intensive organisations depend upon encultured knowledge and collective understandings. However, Blackler also pointed out that it is incorrect to assume that these forms of knowledge are wholly distinct and separate from each other, because knowledge is multi-faceted. Also, as he noted, instead of thinking that knowledge is an 'object' that people have, it is perhaps more useful to regard 'knowing' as something that they do.

Alice Lam (2000) also used Collins' model and, like Blackler, argued that while it is possible to conceptually distinguish between explicit and tacit knowledge, empirically they are rarely completely separate. Nonetheless, like both Blackler and Nonaka, Lam also suggests that in practice, different organisations have different combinations of knowledge types. Tacit knowledge, she notes, is intuitive and unarticulated, and develops from shared understandings and relationships of trust; it is both personal and influenced by context. It is found, in varying degrees, in association with embrained, embodied and embedded knowledge. Lam suggests that there exists a tension between what she terms 'machine bureaucracies' (which rely on encoded knowledge) and other forms of organisation with different dominant forms of knowledge. Therefore in Lam's model, machine bureaucracies attempt to minimise the use of tacit knowledge: they rely upon encoded knowledge, standardisation and control through formalised rules and procedures (Flynn 2002).

Thus, each of these authors notes the dynamic and socially-constructed character of knowledge production and use, and each highlights tensions in the process of transformation between different knowledge types within organisations. The complexity of different ways of conceptualising knowledge types – and the alternative typologies proposed – reflects the complexity of different forms of knowledge in practice. This is significant when we turn to consider attempts to codify professional knowledge and standardise healthcare expertise.

Tacit Knowledge, Expertise and Rule-Based Systems

Various scholars have criticised the normative suggestion that tacit knowledge can – and should be – minimised. The related idea that tacit knowledge can be converted or translated into codified explicit knowledge has also been challenged. Dreyfus and Dreyfus (2005) forcefully argued that expertise generally, and medical expertise specifically, 'cannot be captured in rule-based expert systems, since expertise is based on the making of immediate, unreflective situational responses; intuitive judgement is the hallmark of expertise' (Dreyfus and Dreyfus 2005: 779). D'Eredita and Barreto (2006) tackle the question of whether, and how, tacit knowledge can proliferate within a team. They argue against the notion that tacit knowledge is necessarily personal or 'locked in' an individual's mind. They suggest that tacit knowledge can proliferate, through collaborative interactions and episodes in which knowledge and experience (including 'know-how') is shared. But in this process, codified or explicit knowledge *per se* does not necessarily feature.

Collins (2007) further developed the concept of tacit knowledge by identifying two aspects or forms – 'somatic' tacit knowledge and 'collective' tacit knowledge. The former refers particularly to the intuitive skills required by individuals to accomplish tasks (such as bicycle-riding as in Polanyi's example) and the behavioural properties of human bodies and brains. The latter refers to knowledge which is an emergent property of groups or collectivities, and is the product of experience and socialisation. Applying this to the question of artificial intelligence, Ribeiro and Collins (2007) add further complexity and sophistication. They point out that explicit forms of knowledge 'presuppose shared tacit understandings' (Ribeiro and Collins 2007: 1429). The status of explicit knowledge such as that contained in instruction manuals or books is misleading: it is not comprehensive or exhaustive, and its interpretation and meaning is socially-constructed through use and thus depends on various forms of tacit knowledge.

Experts or professionals conventionally claim autonomy on the basis of a combination of different types of specialised knowledge (Freidson 1994) but often highlight the particular characteristics of tacit knowledge as a vital element in their practice. As Collins and Pinch have shown:

> Knowledge is just one component of expertise. Medical training requires doctors and the like to learn in practice from skilled practitioners – practitioners with experience. This is because many of the skills are tacit and craft-like in character … [D]octors have to learn to deal with the uncertainties of medicine in practice, mastering heuristics, rules of thumb and the other unformalised components of expertise that help them make the correct diagnoses and interventions.

> If information were the same as expertise, then doctors could be replaced by computers, and, assuredly, they cannot. (Collins and Pinch 2005: 219)

Connected with this, and underlining the crucial importance of tacit knowledge for professional experts and expertise, Collins and Evans (2007) proposed a 'Periodic Table of Expertises' in which the idea of tacit knowledge is the chief organising principle. Such tacit knowledge consists of a 'deep understanding' gained from immersion in a social group who already possess it. They emphasise the particular importance of 'ubiquitous expertise', which comprises 'a huge body of tacit knowledge – things you just know how to do without being able to explain the rules for how you do them' (Collins and Evans 2007: 13). This 'inexpressibility' of tacit knowledge makes it very difficult – if not impossible – to formalise or computerise. Specialist and tacit knowledge is acquired through practice and enculturation with a professional team: they suggest it is somewhat similar to learning a natural language. Thus: '"Enculturation" is the only way to master an expertise which is deeply laden with tacit knowledge because it is only through common practice with others that the rules that cannot be written down come to be understood' (Collins and Evans 2007: 24).

The 'craft' component of tacit knowledge has been remarked upon by many other commentators. For Sennett (2008) 'craftsmen [sic] are bearers of embodied knowledge'. Medicine and nursing professionals negotiate 'a liminal zone between problem-solving and problem-finding' (Sennett 2008: 48). Three processes are at work in exercising this craft skill: localising (identifying where something important is happening); questioning (investigating the circumstances and possibilities); and opening-up (using intuition and tacit knowledge to make connections between different domains). This all depends on embedded and embodied (tacit) knowledge. But Sennett (2008) argues that in the British NHS, bureaucratic rationalisers have tried to root out embedded knowledge, and he suggests that the craft element in medicine and nursing is under threat. This tendency reflects a broader current of managerialism – and the threat to professionalism – previously noted by many other commentators (see, for example, Flynn 1992, Gray 2004, Harrison and Ahmed 2000).

Evidence-Based Medicine and Outcome Measures

Attempts to reduce the likelihood of apparently idiosyncratic and inconsistent decision-making in medicine – which were seen as one product of a reliance on individuals' clinical discretion and the use of tacit knowledge – have a long history. They became systematised in many health care systems during the 1980s and were institutionalised as the movement for evidence-based medicine (EBM) discussed in Chapters 1 and 2. This subject matter has received exhaustive attention but some key features should be highlighted. Timmermans and Berg (2003) argued that EBM has not reduced medical uncertainty or the importance of experience in individual decision-making but, rather, it has introduced new types of uncertainties. Clinicians may still vary in applying guidelines, protocols and standards to specific patients or conditions and thus the implementation of EBM is problematic. They observed that clinical experience, which entails an 'almost intuitive sense of appropriate judgement derived from "hands-on" experience' (Timmermans and Berg 2003: 87–8) was challenged by EBM but could not be eliminated by it. While Timmermans and Angel (2001) stressed the interdependency of evidence and experience in clinical judgement, Timmermans and Mauck (2005) suggested that there was a continuing problem of doctors' non-adherence or failure to implement guidelines. Standardisation still only has a tenuous impact on clinical practice (Timmermans and Almeling 2009).

Other researchers have also noted this 'implementation gap', arguing that EBM fails to sufficiently acknowledge the complexity and multi-dimensional nature of clinical decision-making (Dopson et al. 2003, Lambert and Gordon 2006, Waring 2009). Various qualitative studies have illustrated some of the reasons why. Pope (2003) using data from a study of US and UK surgeons, noted that:

> in order to make sense of the unique circumstances of the individual case, doctors used a form of practical knowledge or judgement quite different to the knowledge offered by EBM ... Medicine drew on a more nebulous type of knowledge, variously referred to as 'the other kind of medicine' or the 'grey zones' of clinical practice. (Pope 2003: 273)

Similarly, in their study of doctors and other health care professionals working in primary care groups, Gabbay et al. (2003) showed how processes of collective sense-making were more complex than the linear model used by EBM.

Two important and inter-related elements stand out here. First, concrete and specific medical decisions require the combined use of different types of knowledge, explicit and tacit. Second, medical decision-making rarely resides solely with an individual clinician, and it has an interactional and negotiated character. Information about cases and patient conditions is assembled from different sources; it is also transformed in a social process between different professions. Thus, for example, Berg (1992, 1997) illustrated how physicians mould patients' problems into solvable problems as medical disposals. Diagnosis and treatment entail a translation or transformation process: data are re-constructed to fit particular categories, and there are important routines to facilitate medical action. These locally-situated routines constitute a frame of reference 'encompass[ing] the unwritten rules' for the transformation of data (symptoms) to disposal (treatment) (Berg 1992: 170). By learning these routines, doctors instantaneously comprehend the essential elements of a case. These routines include tried-and-tested procedures, 'what everybody knows and does'. Malterud (1995: 187) similarly commented that medical craftsmanship and clinical judgement required the exercise of intuition and 'experiential, subconscious and unarticulated processes' alongside standardised rules and procedures. Various studies have shown how medical experts must frequently – we would argue inevitably – use both explicit and tacit knowledge. For example, Smith et al.'s (2003) ethnographic study of anaesthetists and operating theatre staff demonstrated how anaesthetists used a variety of types of knowledge simultaneously. They also showed how clinicians believed that 'text-book' knowledge, guidelines and protocols were insufficient for effective practice. Their qualitative data suggested that 'anaesthetics expertise is comprised of a complex balance of explicit and tacit knowledge' (Smith et al. 2003: 327) so that experiential knowledge was necessary to make sense of explicit knowledge.

Similarly, Gabbay and Le May's (2004) ethnographic study of the use of evidence-based guidelines in General Practitioner (GP) practices concluded that:

1. many clinicians were concerned that EBM undervalued the importance of their own tacit knowledge
2. explicit and tacit knowledge was constructed, negotiated and internalised in routine practice
3. individual doctors did not follow the conventional steps of the EBM linear-rational model
4. clinicians rarely consulted guidelines or explicit evidence from research

Gabbay and Le May found that doctors 'relied upon what we have called "mindlines", collectively reinforced, internalised tacit guidelines [informed by many sources and actors] and by other sources of tacit knowledge' (Gabbay and Le May 2004: 1014). These mindlines might be modified when applied to individual patients and underwent negotiation during consultations; they had a contingent, provisional and iterative quality. Such mindlines encapsulated tacit and explicit knowledge, and, Gabbay and Le May argue, they were more complex than 'heuristics', 'rules-of-thumb' or clinical protocols. They describe mindlines as internalised guidelines which cannot be reduced to codified knowledge. Quinlan (2009) has reported similar findings about the importance of tacit knowledge in primary care teams, but also showed how it led to the development of new explicit knowledge. This resonates with the theoretical analysis of the relationship between tacit and explicit knowledge suggested (and referred to above) by Blackler, Lam and Nonaka.

Others have argued that despite the widespread diffusion of EBM, its practice is mediated by many different factors. Individual clinicians – albeit working within teams – still have to make highly personalised decisions in selecting which components of evidence to act upon, and how to treat their individual patients. Cambrosio et al. (2006) have described how a system of regulatory objectivity has permeated biomedicine and modern health care systems but it has not changed the unalterable reality that doctors, using clinical judgement, 'always evaluated different types of evidence on an individual and informal basis' (Cambrosio et al. 2006: 195). Medicine practised in different contexts will necessarily require different mixtures of explicit and tacit knowledge. Thus, May et al. (2006)

contrast two types of medical knowledge: experimental evidence from RCTs, population studies and meta-analyses; and experiential understanding based on clinical encounters. May et al. suggest that these two types of knowledge are in tension and particularly problematic when applied in the shared decision-making commonly required in primary care. They argue that standardisation and clinical guidelines do not always fit neatly with the exigencies of everyday GP practices where patient expectations and preferences are increasingly seen as important in a consumer encounter. Nettleton et al.'s (2008) intensive qualitative study of the working lives of 47 NHS doctors found that different aspects of modernisation and regulation were contributing to the erosion of tacit knowledge and the disembodiment of medicine. But despite (or because of?) this, 'doctors value experiential, tactic and hands-on knowledge and practice' – what we here regard as 'embodied' and embedded knowledge – and use this to supplement encoded and formal knowledge' (Nettleton et al. 2008: 345).

In summary, EBM seeks to reduce arbitrariness and variation in medical decision-making, but the use of clinical guidelines and protocols is always likely to be incomplete and constrained because of variability in individual patients and their conditions, and because individual clinicians will vary in the degree to which they selectively use explicit or encoded knowledge and tacit or embodied knowledge.

Outcome Measurement and Clinical Interpretation in Neurorehabilitation

To illustrate how this might affect judgements about health outcomes for patients, this section presents qualitative data about clinicians' uses of standardised outcome measures in the field of neurorehabilitation. First we briefly outline the character and purpose of health outcome measures (OMs) generally, and then describe the particular OMs used in neurorehabilitation. Health outcome measures have been identified as crucial components of evidence-based medicine: outcome measures are supposed to show whether there has been a change (improvement or deterioration) in a patient's condition as a result of medical intervention. There are a wide range of health outcome measures used to evaluate treatment effectiveness. The majority of these OMs have been developed on the basis of large-scale quantitative studies either using specialised tests carried out by healthcare practitioners (of patient functions) or questionnaires administered to patients to self-assess their health or quality of life. According to the United Kingdom NHS National Centre for Health Outcomes Development (NHS NCHOD), health outcome measures indicate changes in health, health-related status, or risk factors affecting health (NHS NCHOD, no date). Usually OMs are expressed in a numerical score. They represent an explicit baseline (or even a target) against which the impact of treatment can be assessed. By definition, they represent, but are also derived from, codified and systematic evidence-based knowledge. While there are many different outcome measures available for different types of conditions, there is considerable uncertainty about how extensively they are used, or indeed, how they are used by clinicians and whether they have a significant influence on medical decisions (Greenhalgh et al. 2005).

To examine clinicians' interpretation of OMs in practice, a qualitative case-study of neurorehabilitation was undertaken. Neurorehabilitation was selected for four main reasons: first, there are well-established standardised outcome measures in widespread use; second, neurorehabilitation patients often have severe and multiple impairments (such as cognitive and physical impairments usually following traumatic brain injury, stroke or multiple sclerosis) that demand a range of treatments so assessments of change in a patient's condition are especially important; third, neurorehabilitation is a speciality which involves a multi-disciplinary team where different professions make assessments and recommendations for treatment that are linked with particular outcome measures (Parry 2009); and fourth, it was assumed that as neurorehabilitation is at the interface between acute and community care and thus that outcome measures might be crucial in determining whether a patient can be discharged to their own home or to long-term nursing and residential care outside of a hospital setting with its additional resource implications.

In neurorehabilitation, a number of outcome measures are commonly used. One of the most extensively used is the Barthel Index, but others are also used. Sometimes OMs are used in combination; for example the Functional Independence Measure (FIM) and Functional Assessment Measure (FAM) are often used in conjunction with one another as are the Northwick Park Dependency Score and the Nottingham Extended Activities of Daily Living Scale. Each of these OMs represent a way of measuring a patient's capability for various activities required for daily living (Greenhalgh et al. 2008a, 2008b, Tyson et al. 2010). In general, they indicate the patient's degree of dependence and the extent to which they need continuous care. Specifically, they inform decision making as to whether the patient can be discharged to their own home with community health services support or whether they will require continuing care in a residential or nursing unit. The Barthel Index is a clinician-rated composite measure based on a standardised questionnaire which assesses a variety of factors that include the patient's bowel and bladder control (continence); their ability to wash, bathe, dress and carry out other personal care; their ability to feed themselves; whether they can transfer from a bed to a chair or to a wheelchair; their overall mobility and whether they can use stairs. Scores given for each of these items are estimates and an overall score (usually out of a total of 100, but in some versions, 20) is recorded, where zero indicates complete dependence and 100 indicates complete independence. The Barthel Index is therefore one example of a very specific type of explicit and encoded knowledge.

A qualitative study was conducted that investigated the use of outcome measures in one English National Health Service neurorehabilitation (in-patient) unit (further details about methods, and other findings may be found in Greenhalgh et al. 2008a, 2008b, Tyson et al. 2010). Non-participant observation and semi-structured interviewing was carried out together with documentary analysis. Sixteen of the regular meetings of the multi-disciplinary team (MDT) were attended and observed, and audio-recorded. In this period, 39 different patients were discussed. After the observation of team meetings had been completed, semi-structured interviews were conducted with the clinicians including the consultants, the registrar, the senior house officer (SHO) and other team members – the specialist nurse, physiotherapist, occupational therapist (OT), speech and language therapist (SALT), social worker and health visitor. The MDT meetings had a formal character, with an agenda, supporting documentation and booklets available that contained scoring guidelines for the outcome measures. Two consultants presided over these meetings and clinical practitioners considered a number of patients (usually six or seven) at each meeting, which lasted one-and-a-half to two hours.

The qualitative data analysis highlighted several processes: the ways in which individual clinicians appeared to decide on the scores; the ways in which the MDT collectively discussed and debated those scores for particular patients; and the ways in which the Barthel Index (and other outcome measures) were used in decisions about further treatment or discharge. We present selected illustrations of the uses of tacit knowledge observed in the MDT meetings and reflections by research participants in subsequent interviews.

Overall, a number of features seemed to underlie the meetings. First, during the MDT meetings, the discussion of each case had a ritualistic character, much as other researchers have shown (Anspach 1998, Atkinson 1995, Strong 1979) with each clinician reading out or reciting 'their' scores for particular patients. Second, it was difficult to determine when a decision had been reached by the MDT, as there was hardly ever any explicit acknowledgement, following consideration of the Barthel scores, of whether agreement had been reached as to a specific course of action for each patient. The implications for future action seemed to be unspoken or taken-for-granted. Again, this echoes findings from other ethnographers who have noted that in practice it is sometimes difficult to identify a concrete decision (Hughes and Griffiths 1997). Third, in the process of case-presentation, a narrative of the patient (and their family) was constructed by the clinicians to supplement – and sometimes to challenge – the scores. The clinical judgements about the facts of the case were also implicitly linked with, and amplified by, moral evaluations about the patients' personal and home circumstances (Atkinson 1995, Brookes-Howell 2006, White and Stancombe 2003).

From the observations of the MDT, it was evident that everybody seemed to know what the Barthel Index scores meant, or represented. There were few instances in which a particular clinician's score was challenged or questioned by others, though discussions about what the score should be did occur (Greenhalgh et al. 2008b). What prompted discussion was the implication of the score, whether it entailed no change in the patient's condition, or sufficient improvement for discharge. The score alone often did not provide sufficient information to determine whether a patient could go home, other information was necessary to contextualise the scores. For example, in the first MDT meeting observed, discussion of Patient 1 included debate about whether the patient had 'confusion', poor concentration and memory. The Consultant and SALT agreed that it was hard to assess the degree of confusion, and the OT said it was also hard to assess memory. Thus:

Registrar 1:	Confusion?
Occupational Therapist 1:	I think it's hard to assess it really, because he's not quite … […]
Consultant 1:	Or does anybody think he's normal?
Speech and Language Therapist:	It's hard to tell …
Consultant 1:	Yes it is, isn't it.
Registrar 1:	Concentration?
Occupational Therapist 1:	Erm, … I would say probably four.
Registrar 1:	Memory?
Occupational Therapist 1:	Again it's hard to assess.

This extract shows that scoring was difficult because it was hard to tell whether the patient had memory/cognitive or speech problems. If someone cannot speak, it is hard to tell whether they are understanding things. The speech therapist (during an interview) emphasised this:

> sometimes if people have dysphasia it's quite hard to tell whether they've got memory problems and confusion and things because it's just hard to assess when somebody can't find the right words you don't know whether it's a word finding problem or that they're confused.

What this also illustrates is that producing the scores fundamentally depends on the team's working knowledge of the patient, their tacit knowledge. As Consultant 1 noted in an interview:

> the one thing the Barthel doesn't do is tell you anything about cognitive function, it does indirectly because he can't dress because he can't think about the neglect or the shape of your t-shirt you're putting on but it gives you no real idea of cognitive function and that's a huge determining factor.

Thus, although the scores might have the appearance of 'objectivising' certain forms of knowledge about the patient this is limited to (and limited by) the extent of the clinicians' tacit knowledge. In this instance, further information about the patient was necessary to make any decision about their likely discharge destination. This led to a further discussion of the raw scores pertaining to the possibility of sending the patient to their own home. Questions were asked about the patient's family circumstances and social background: a home visit and meeting with the family was deemed necessary. Scores by themselves were insufficient; they required explication and additional information to render them meaningful.

Frequently there was debate about possible changes in a patient's condition and whether the scores accurately measured these. There was some recognition that scores were influenced by the clinicians' greater familiarity with the patient. For example, discussion of Patient 14 (MDT meeting 3), who had significant cognitive problems as a result of a head injury, prompted considerable deliberation about the appropriateness of the Barthel scores. This was the end of this patient's second week after admission and the second time he had been scored. Thus:

Registrar 2:	[Patient 14]? So, erm, his scores? Transfer, ambulation – zero I presume still?
Physiotherapist 2:	Yeah, all the same.
Registrar 2:	Erm, feeding – scored two here. Dressing – still zero?

[Occupational Therapist and Physiotherapist consult scoring guidelines]

Registrar 2:	Two it is. Personal hygiene?
Occupational Therapist:	Erm, a one, oh, sorry, zero …
Registrar 2:	Erm, I think we may have been guessing last week, so we score him one.
Consultant:	Yeah. Erm, I mean, I think that this is indicating getting to know him, rather than any deterioration.

This dialogue suggests that where the clinicians' tacit knowledge and the explicit knowledge indicated by the scores were at odds, tacit knowledge was used to adjust or dismiss the scores. Further, this indicates that the initial score was fundamentally dependent on the clinicians' knowledge of the patient (their tacit knowledge) and that this was incomplete at the time of the patient's admission and thus initial scores were inaccurate in the light of new information (Greenhalgh et al. 2008b). Although the initial scores formalised the available tacit knowledge about the patient's cognitive problems, in producing a score on admission clinicians skilfully used their tacit knowledge to re-evaluate the accuracy of this now formalised explicit knowledge (the score) in light of new information about the patient.

A degree of indeterminacy about the scoring, and the malleability of the scores themselves, was also observed in MDT discussions. At a later MDT meeting, a new patient (Patient 18) was reviewed: each team member recited their scores, and at one point the guidelines were checked. During this discussion, medical students were present, and the consultant, addressing them, highlighted some caveats surrounding the Barthel Index. The consultant suggested that the initial score was a 'pot shot'. There was some disagreement about the scoring for orientation and social integration, with some divergence between the Registrar and the SALT. The consultant commented that there was a low Barthel but a high handicap score and she advised that they should 'mark him down'. This reflects the view that where there was uncertainty about the patient's condition, a low score allowed an opportunity to measure subsequent improvement. At several other meetings, and in connection with other patients, scores were adjusted during the case-conference, after the patient's goals had been reviewed and also in the context of information about the extent of family support, domestic arrangements and social services provision. Thus the scores in themselves, as part of the clinical assessment, were mediated by inter-professional judgements and also influenced by external factors; similar findings have been noted elsewhere (Dixon-Woods et al. 2009, Gross 2009, Kontos and Naglie 2009). Here again, explicit and encoded knowledge was elaborated by other forms of (implicit) knowledge.

Uncertainties surrounding the outcome measures also surfaced at a later MDT meeting over Patient 8. This particular patient's wife was also seriously ill and unable to care for him, and his house would have to be modified if he was discharged to his own home. Clinicians compared scores and also referred to the booklet containing scoring guidelines in order to check the criteria. The consultant alluded to the inadequacy of some of the Barthel Index scores and difficulty in relating them to practical aspects of discharging patients. She asked medical students attending the meeting:

> Can you see, when you deal with somebody who is a whole person, inside a family, you get a picture which you need?

The inference here was that the apparently objective scores had to be interpreted and placed within a wider context, necessitating other types of information, not all of which was measurable or even known.

In the same meeting, discussing Patient 12, clinicians listed their own scores, and the consultant then asked medical students if these indicated a discharge home. She noted that, although the Northwick Park Dependency score suggested the patient needed 'a fair amount of help', other factors were also relevant. She asked the medical students: 'OK, does the Barthel tell you anything about him as a person? Did you get any feel for him as a person?' Following the students' comments, the consultant affirmed that the Barthel did not give them the 'feel' of the person, and that other methods of assessment were needed. In later discussion directed at the medical students, the consultant observed that:

> the form of the [MDT] meeting is structured but I think there is a certain amount of intuitive decision-making going on, just because you are weighing up all the variations on information, and which one is higher in the hierarchy that affects that particular person. So it's mostly quite skilled.

This allusion to 'the feel' for the patient again reveals the significance of embodied, embedded and tacit knowledge.

The importance of tacit knowledge and uses of intuition also became apparent in the interviews with clinicians. For example, Consultant 2 was very reflexive about the limitations of outcome measures, noting that OMs cannot be the only way of measuring how a patient progresses. She remarked:

> I think it's based on a mixture of seeing no change in the scores, and clinical experience and expertise. It certainly shouldn't be one without the other because you know, the scores are not infallible. ... We know that they have limitations in terms of sensitivity and specificity ... so you can't rely on a single measure. ... [It] has to be tempered with clinical experience.

Similarly, the speech and language therapist, asked to explain how different therapists in the MDT deal with the scores, commented that:

> I think the team do use them [Barthel and other OMs] to that extent, but equally they'll just come up to me and talk to me about it rather than running off the scores, I think because, you know, they [the scores] don't pick up the subtleties do they?

The specialist rehabilitation nurse emphasised the many different factors involved in making a discharge decision, commenting that the total Barthel score was inadequate by itself: '*We ourselves know whether the patient's improved* [authors' emphasis] from week to week, but that's [Barthel score] just going to put down on paper that the patient has improved'. The occupational therapist acknowledged some of the limitations of outcome measures, but also indicated their positive uses:

> It's very subjective, but then I think it's not a quantitative thing, is it? It's qualitative ... It's [Barthel Index] not the be-all and end-all, it never can be and it never will. But it, the objectives, do help for measuring if there are changes, or if there are not, then it can start the process of questioning.

A more critical view emerged from a recently appointed specialist registrar, who expressed difficulty in understanding the meaning of the outcome measures and significance of the scores. He stressed the necessity of using tacit knowledge in making clinical decisions:

> People who are clinically, you know, professional, and say 'Look this person doesn't need [this treatment] and the score is maybe keeping at that'. But I don't think that really influences it. To be honest, there are people with their own clinical experience and their own judgement, you know, and they form their own impression, a decision to say 'Yes this person [needs treatment]'. You look at the scores: I suppose they don't add anything from certainly our perspective anyway.

This doctor then went on to refer to using a 'feel factor' to 'perfect' the scores. He also commented that such scores had a broader instrumental purpose:

demonstrating to the hospital trust management and the patient's family that treatment was making a difference. In evaluating whether a patient was making progress, he insisted that 'you go on your clinical impression, you know, *your feeling* if you want to call it that, rather than the score' [authors' emphasis].

A very similar view was expressed by a senior house officer. Responding to an interview question about whether she had gone through any training in the unit on the use of the Barthel guidelines, she noted that they had been taught about it previously, but had to become familiar with the protocol: '*using it comes from doing it* rather than being told what to do' [authors' emphasis]. She went on to recognise the usefulness of scores as a guide to treatment, but also acknowledged that:

> from day to day, erm, again it's quite good just to look at it as a snapshot. But in terms of, you know, how you decide ongoing treatment … I think that's probably done better, erm, from direct experience.

These interviews indicate that while the medical professionals and other health care practitioners routinely used the Barthel Index and other standardised outcome measures, they did so in a contingent and flexible way. They adjusted the scores when other types of information were available. For example, this additional information was derived from observations of or encounters with patients on the ward (rather than when administering the tests for example) or judgements after meetings with family members. This type of information was not formalised or even necessarily officially recorded; it was certainly not encoded and arguably was incapable of being encoded. The interviews also display these clinicians' endorsement of the validity of their subjective experience and intuitive understanding of the patient and other similar or previous cases, which underlies both their own and their colleagues' embodied and embedded knowledge.

Conclusions

We acknowledge the specificity of this qualitative case study, and the need for further research to explore these processes in greater depth. However, we suggest that our findings have broader relevance. The particular unit selected was typical of similar units in the English NHS, and the cases (types of patient and condition) treated were also broadly typical. The outcome measures are officially regarded as valid and reliable, and are in constant and general use in the UK and internationally. We argue that the qualitative data reported here give valuable insights into the process of clinical decision-making using outcome measures and are convergent with findings from similar recent ethnographic studies (cf. Gross 2009, Kontos and Naglie 2009, Parry 2009). In particular, the case-study material shows the simultaneous and parallel uses of encoded or technical knowledge, and implicit or tacit knowledge. It also indicates how decision-making within a multi-professional team necessarily involves a deliberative and negotiated form of clinical judgement, rather than simple rule-following or application of a standardised protocol.

This study provides further evidence in support of Polanyi's (1966) insistence on the ineffaceable and inevitable nature of tacit knowledge. It also illustrates Blackler's (1995) and Lam's (2000) observations that professional expertise comprises a mixture of different types of knowledge – embrained, embodied, embedded and encoded. But what is also evident is that in neurorehabilitation, health care practitioners become enculturated or socialised into a particular form of what Collins (2007) has described as collective tacit knowledge. Health care practitioners employ tacit craft skills (Collins and Pinch 2005) to interpret the outcome measures and to determine the most appropriate treatment for their patients. But some writers, such as Sennett (2008) have argued that in contemporary society, this 'craftsmanship' is threatened by standardisation and routinisation, and that this threat is becoming ever more prevalent within health care systems. Flynn (2004) argued that NHS medical professionals' expertise is being undermined by regulatory procedures usually associated with machine-bureaucracies. This case-study suggests that, however well-intentioned and desirable it may be to employ the systematic procedures contained within evidence-based medicine, there are limits on the practical implementation of guidelines, rules and protocols. The encoded knowledge represented by health outcome measures is necessarily mediated by professional expertise and judgement, and constantly interpreted (and re-interpreted) using tacit knowledge.

Evidence-based medicine (and the use of protocols for evidence-based heathcare) is likely to continue and expand to cover an ever-widening variety of clinical specialties and treatments. Patient groups, insurers, professional bodies and government regulators are increasingly likely to demand greater standardisation of performance by health care workers and professionals. While these demands and pressures are understandable, the evidence from this small-scale study (as well as others) shows that many of the essential decisions and tasks undertaken by medical and nursing staff routinely involve – and indeed may actually require – the use of tacit knowledge. To seek to reduce it, or eliminate it, risks undermining some of the defining features of professional and clinical judgement with the potential result being increased uncertainty in outcomes for all involved.

Acknowledgements

The study on which this chapter is based was funded by the ESRC (RES-000-22-1117).We also wish to acknowledge the co-operation of the (anonymous) NHS Trust for giving access for the research, and to the staff for their help. The project had NHS and university ethical approval. The study design was collaborative between team members; all the fieldwork and data collection was undertaken by Joanne Greenhalgh; all members of the team participated in qualitative data analysis.

References

Anspach, R. 1998. Notes on the sociology of medical discourse: The language of case-presentation. *Journal of Health and Social Behavior*, 29(4), 357–75.

Atkinson, P. 1995. *Medical Talk and Medical Work: The Liturgy of the Clinic*. London: Sage.

Berg, M. 1992 The construction of medical disposals: Medical sociology and medical problem-solving in clinical practice. *Sociology of Health and Illness*, 14(2), 151–80.

Bittner, E. 1974. The concept of organization, in *Ethnomethodology*, edited by R. Turner. Harmondsworth: Penguin.

Blackler, F. 1995. Knowledge, knowledge work and organizations: An overview and an interpretation. *Organization Studies*, 16(6), 1021–46.

Brookes-Howell, L. 2006. Living without labels: The interactional management of diagnostic uncertainty in the genetic counselling clinic. *Social Science and Medicine*, 63, 3080–91.

Cambrosio, A., Keating, P., Schlick, T. and Weisz, G. 2006. Regulatory objectivity and the generation and management of evidence in medicine. *Social Science and Medicine*, 63, 189–99.

Collins, H. and Evans, R. 2007. *Rethinking Expertise*. Chicago and London: University of Chicago Press.

Collins, H. 2007. Bicycling on the moon: Collective tacit knowledge and somatic-limit tacit knowledge. *Organization Studies*, 28(2), 257–62.

Collins, H. and Pinch, T. 2005. *Dr Golem: How to Think About Medicine*. Chicago and London: University of Chicago Press.

Collins, H.M. 1993. The structure of knowledge. *Social Research*, 60(1), 95–116.

D'Eredita, M. and Barreto, C. 2006. How does tacit knowledge proliferate? *Organization Studies*, 27(12), 1821–41.

Dixon-Woods, M., Suokas, A., Pitchforth, E. and Tarrant, C. 2009. An ethnographic study of classifying and accounting for risk at the sharp end of medical wards. *Social Science and Medicine*, 69, 362–9.

Dopson, S., Locock, L., Gabbay, J., Ferlie, E. and Fitzgerald, L. 2003. Evidence-based medicine and the implementation gap. *Health*, 7(3), 311–30.

Dreyfus, H. and Dreyfus, S. 2005. Expertise in real world contexts. *Organization Studies*, 26(5), 779–92.

Flynn, R. 1992. *Structures of Control in Health Management*. London: Routledge.

Flynn, R. 2002. Clinical governance and governmentality. *Health, Risk and Society*, 4(2), 155–73.

Flynn, R. 2004. 'Soft bureaucracy', governmentality and clinical governance, in *Governing Medicine*, edited by A. Gray and S. Harrison. Maidenhead: Open University Press.

Freidson, E. 1994. *Professionalism Reborn*. Cambridge: Polity Press.

Gabbay, J. and LeMay, A. 2004. Evidence-based guidelines or collectively-constructed 'mindlines': Ethnographic study of knowledge management in primary care. *British Medical Journal*, 329, 1013.

Gabbay, J., LeMay, A., Jefferson, H., Webb, D., Lovelock, R., Powell, J. and Lathlean, J. 2003. A case-study of knowledge-based management in multi-agency consumer-informed communities of practice. *Health*, 7(3), 283–310.

Gray, A. 2004. Governing medicine: An introduction, in *Governing Medicine*, edited by A. Gray and S. Harrison. Maidenhead: Open University Press.

Greenhalgh, J., Flynn, R., Long, A.F. and Tyson, S. 2008a. Tacit and encoded knowledge in the use of standardised outcome measures in multi-disciplinary team decision-making: A case-study in neurorehabilitation. *Social Science and Medicine*, 67, 183–94.

Greenhalgh, J, Long, A.F., Flynn, R. and Tyson, S. 2008b. 'It's hard to tell': The challenges of scoring patients on standardised outcome measures by multi-disciplinary teams – A case-study of neurorehabilitation. *BMC Health Services Research*, 8, 217–37. [Online]. Available at: http://www.biomedcentral.com/1472-6963/8/217 [accessed: 9 October 2009].

Greenhalgh, J., Long, A.F. and Flynn, R. 2005. The use of patient-reported outcome measures in routine clinical practice. *Social Science and Medicine*, 60, 833–43.

Gross, S. 2009. Experts and 'knowledge that counts': A study into the world of brain cancer diagnosis. *Social Science and Medicine*, 69, 1819–26.

Harrison, S. and Ahmad, W. 2000. Medical autonomy and the UK state 1975 to 2025. *Sociology*, 34(1), 129–46.

Hughes, D. and Griffiths, L. 1997. 'Ruling-in' and 'ruling-out': Two approaches to the micro-rationing of health care. *Social Science and Medicine*, 44(5), 589–99.

Kontos, P. and Naglie, G. 2009. Tacit knowledge of caring and embodied selfhood. *Sociology of Health and Illness*, 31(5), 688–704.

Lam, A. 2000. Tacit knowledge, organizational learning and societal institutions: An integrated framework. *Organization Studies*, 21(3), 487–513.

Lambert, H. 2006 Accounting for EBM: Notions of evidence in medicine. *Social Science and Medicine*, 62, 2633–45.

Lambert, H. and Gordon, E. 2006. Gift horse or Trojan horse? Social science perspectives on evidence-based health care. *Social Science and Medicine*, 62, 2613–20.

Malterud, K. 1995. The legitimacy of clinical knowledge: Towards a medical epistemology embracing the art of medicine. *Theoretical Medicine*, 16, 183–98.

May, C., Rapley, T., Moreira, T., Finch, T. and Heaven, B. 2006. Technogovernance, evidence, subjectivity and the clinical encounter in primary care medicine. *Social Science and Medicine*, 62, 1022–30.

Nettleton, S., Burrows, R. and Watt, I. 2008. Regulating medical bodies? The modernisation of the NHS and the disembodiment of clinical knowledge. *Sociology of Health and Illness*, 30(2), 333–48.

NHS NCHOD (no date) *Clinical and Health Outcomes Knowledge Base, Concepts and Frameworks: Definitions*. National Centre for Health Outcomes

Development. Available at: http://www.nchod.nhs.uk/NCHOD/HomeDb2R6.
nsf [accessed: 6 June 2008].

Nonaka, I. 1994. A dynamic theory of organizational knowledge creation. *Organization Science*, 5(1), 14–37.

Nonaka, I. and van Krogh, G. 2009. Tacit knowledge and knowledge conversion: Controversy and advancement in organizational knowledge creation theory. *Organization Science*, 20(3), 635–52.

Parry, R. 2009. Practitioners' accounts for treatment actions and recommendations in physiotherapy: When do they occur, how are they structured, and what do they do? *Sociology of Health and Illness*, 31(6), 835–53.

Polanyi, M. 1958. *Personal Knowledge*. London: Routledge and Kegan Paul.

Polanyi, M. 1983. *The Tacit Dimension*. Gloucester: Peter Smith [Original work published 1966].

Pope, C. 2003. Resisting evidence: The study of evidence-based medicine as a contemporary social movement. *Health*, 7(3), 267–82.

Quinlan, E. 2009. The 'actualities' of knowledge work: An institutional ethnography of multi-disciplinary primary health care team. *Sociology of Health and Illness*, 31(5), 625–41.

Ribeiro, R. and Collins, H. 2007. The bread-making machine: Tacit knowledge and two types of action. *Organization Studies*, 28(9), 1417–33.

Sennett, R. 2008. *The Craftsman*. London: Allen Lane.

Smith, A., Goodwin, D., Mort, M. and Pope, C. 2003. Expertise in practice: An ethnographic study exploring acquisition and use of knowledge in anaesthesia. *British Journal of Anaesthesia*, 91(3), 319–28.

Strong, P. 1979. *The Ceremonial Order of the Clinic*. London: Routledge and Kegan Paul.

Timmermans, S. and Almeling, R. 2009. Objectification, standardization and commodification in health care: A conceptual readjustment. *Social Science and Medicine*, 69, 21–7.

Timmermans, S. and Mauck, A. 2005. The promises and pitfalls of evidence-based medicine. *Health Affairs*, 24, 18–28.

Timmermans, S. and Angell, A. 2001. Evidence-based medicine, clinical uncertainty and learning to doctor. *Journal of Health and Social Behavior*, 42(4), 342–59.

Timmermans, S. and Berg, M. 2003. *The Gold Standard*. Philadelphia: Temple University Press.

Tyson, S., Greenhalgh, J., Long, A.F. and Flynn, R. 2010. The use of measurement tools in clinical practice: An observational study of neurorehabilitation. *Clinical Rehabilitation*, 24, 74–81.

Waring, J. 2009. Constructing and re-constructing narratives of patient safety. *Social Science and Medicine*, 69, 1722–31.

White, S. and Stancombe, J. 2003. *Clinical Judgement in the Health and Welfare Professions*. Maidenhead: Open University Press.

Chapter 6

The Histories and Cultures of Evidence Utilisation: The Cases of Medical Oncology and Haematology

Alex Broom and Jon Adams

Introduction

As outlined in our introduction to this book, the idea of EBM or EBP, for biomedical clinicians, is to apply the best evidence to the clinical condition they are presented with. However, while EBM may seem to be mere commonsense, in actuality, and particularly in the context of specialties like medical oncology and haematology, it presents a plethora of ideological, epistemological and practical issues. We argue here that for oncology clinicians operating at a grassroots level there is often a disconnection between EBM (and processes of standardisation) and the actual character of contemporary oncological work (De Vries and Lemmens 2006). Furthermore, the very value judgements and subjectivities that often go unrecognised in an EBM framework are actually critically important skills in oncology and haematology practice (Tredaniel et al. 2005). In oncology such disjunctions are accentuated with the constant development of new interventions (Ioannidis, Schmid and Lau 2000) combined with the omnipresent need to 'try new things' with potentially terminal patients where standard treatments do not work.

As outlined in Chapter 1, increased standardisation can produce a conflict between *res ipsa loquitur* ('the thing speaks for itself') and objective scientific evidence in any given medical context. This tension between what *is* happening and what *should* be happening is greatly enhanced in oncology as the reality of the patient dying while receiving chemotherapy (which was statistically likely to cure them) can be hard to reconcile with the clinical evidence available (Cox 2000). The focus on evidence and standardisation is ultimately partnered with a diminishment in acceptance (or allowance of) the diagnostic art or clinical judgement, thus silencing the individual clinician and the patient by simultaneously suppressing the role of illness narratives and the 'expert eye' in medical work (Greenhalgh 1999). As Goldenberg (2006) suggests, an EBM framework tends to ignore the phenomenology of illness; the embodied, experiential facets of being treated (the patient experience) and treating (the doctor's experience). Given these issues it is perhaps unsurprising that EBM is not always well received and can be difficult to actualise in oncology contexts (De Vries and Lemmens 2006, Lambert 2006). Exactly how differently positioned oncology[1] clinicians manage the practice of EBM; how they utilise forms of expertise in clinical practice; and, how they augment this with clinical intuition is largely unknown. As such, in this chapter we focus on how EBM is shaping experiences of medical work more broadly in oncology, its impacts on organisational hierarchies and expertise, and the experiences of different sub-specialities within oncology.

Histories of Oncology

In thinking about EBM and the mediation of evidence in Australian medical oncology and haematology, some reflection on the historical trajectories of these sub-specialities is useful. Firstly, it must be recognised that the historical trajectory of medical oncology is closely tied to the history of the discovery and development of chemotherapy. Although targeted drugs are now being developed and radiation oncology is an increasingly critical element of medical oncology practice, traditional chemotherapy regimens still remain a central part of everyday oncological work and a defining element of its historical trajectory (Chabner and Roberts 2005). The treatment of solid tumours, and thus development of medical oncology as a sub-specialty, was greatly influenced by the development of various chemotherapeutic agents in the second half of the twentieth century (including cisplatin and paclitaxel) which showed promising activity in a range of solid tumours (Chabner and Roberts 2005). However, initial expectations of chemotherapy development resulted in a tendency to over-treat, with a focus on pushing patients to the brink of death and then pulling them back (Davidson 2007). Due to a continued lack of success in many solid tumours relative to toxicity, medical oncology gradually moved away from a largely interventionalist approach involving acute toxicity to a focus on chronic care (that is, towards a focus on remission or containment) (Davidson 2007).

The historic trajectory of haematological oncology is quite different to that of medical oncology in terms of the various successes responsible for shaping public and medical perception. Although key advances were made in the 1940s with nitrogen mustard, it was between 1965 and 1975, with the advent of combination chemotherapy for inducing long-term remissions in children with acute lymphoblastic leukaemia (ALL), that significant advances were made. Alongside advances in the treatment of ALL, Vincent DeVita and colleagues also cured lymphomas with combination chemotherapy (both non-Hodgkin's and Hodgkin's) (Chabner and Roberts 2005). Whilst advances in treating solid tumours emerged concurrently, they were generally not as dramatic as those seen in haematology, particularly in the context of childhood malignancies. As such,

---

1   From here on in, 'oncology' is used to refer to both medical oncology and haematological oncology.

in the current study we were interested in exploring whether the character and histories of these medical sub-specialties shaped their mediation of evidence and perspectives on EBM.

The Emergence of Evidence-Based Nursing Practice (EBNP)

Oncology practice is ultimately a team-based activity with allied health, nursing, medicine and social work all feeding into patient care. While moves to standardise professions (and their practices) has moved well beyond medicine (incorporating physiotherapy, psychology and social work), EBNP represents an important case study of the extension of EBM into multiple spheres of the healthcare workforce. It is also particularly interesting given the differences between EBM and EBNP in terms of ideology and purpose.

In the wider context of the nursing profession, EBM has played an important, albeit at times problematic role in nursing professionalisation with EBNP gaining significant strength over the last decade. However, whilst EBM frameworks have posed difficulties for doctors in terms of individual autonomy, for nursing the problematic of EBM is centred on the commensurability of abstracted models of patient care and nursing work (Kessenich, Guyatt and DiCenso 1997). Whilst nursing has drawn heavily on the principles of EBM for professionalisation purposes, this process has also involved a trajectory of ideological and methodological distinction from medicine (Tovey and Adams 2003); a multifaceted process of professional delineation that is fundamentally shaping its representation; and, to a lesser extent, enactment of EBNP in oncology nursing. Specifically, the absorption of EBM may be contested by the desire to retain or pursue distinction from medicine through an emphasis on the 'true origins' of nursing practice (for example, holism, empowerment and patient centredness) and some degree of resistance to a pursuit of a purely biomedical view of healing (Boschma 1994, Helms 2006, Light 1997). To date, little is known about how these processes may manifest in oncology nurses' accounts of EBM.

In developing this study we set out to examine conceptions about evidence in the Australian oncology context with a focus on medical specialist and nursing perspectives. How would EBM be viewed in an area of medicine dealing with the imminent threat of terminality and individual trauma? How would EBM be viewed where the importance of certainty (given potential toxicity) is paramount? What would be the impact of EBM within a medico-political context of a pressure to treat and how would best-practice and the various manifestations of EBM fit with the highly contingent issues dealt with in oncology work such as survival benefit, quality of life and chances of cure? Finally, how do individual oncology departments respond to the challenges of the rationalisation of care and the desires and actions of individual clinicians?

Fieldwork

We selected the two main hospitals that provide cancer services in a state capital in Australia. Both provide care for solid tumour (medical oncology) cancers and haematological malignancies. After ethics approval was secured from both hospitals, we approached hospital management regarding participation of the oncology/haematology consultants and nurses. Agreement was reached and clinicians in both hospitals were informed about the study via email. In total, 25 clinicians participated in a 45–60 minute in-depth interview, including several who had academic roles in local universities. We interviewed 13 medical specialists (consultant medical oncologists and haematological oncologists) and 12 medical oncology/haematology nurses. We included a spread of ages, seniority and involvement in research and academia to ensure heterogeneity in the sample. The interviews explored: the nature of evidence and clinical effectiveness; how clinicians view, utilise and translate evidence in their everyday work; how evidence relates to grassroots clinical practice; and, the benefits and challenges of evidence-based medicine within oncology. Examples of the questions asked include: What constitutes evidence in your perspective? What is the relationship between evidence and clinical effectiveness in oncology/haematology? What constitutes evidence-based medicine or evidence-based nursing and how do such notions feed into or shape clinical practice?

What is Evidence? Balancing Theory, Study Design and What is in Front of You

The interviews began with an examination of the finer points of what constituted evidence for the individual clinician in their organisational context. The intention was to begin the interviews by examining the assumptive basis of wider 'talk' of evidence-based medicine and evidence-based practice. Whilst there was a degree of consensus regarding definitions, there was also considerable differentiation:

Clinician: [A study] doesn't necessarily have to be randomised evidence for
                [the treatment] to be used clinically. Although that's preferable.
Interviewer: … but at what point do you consider something to be effective?
Clinician: Well I guess there being some evidence that it actually works.
Interview: How do you know it works?
Clinician: Because the patient gets better. (Medical oncologist)

Another respondent:
Interviewer: In your view, what is evidence?
Clinician: Evidence is a … um, [a] study which has been published in
                a peer-reviewed journal or presented at an international meeting,
                or the drug which has gone through the standard assessment. It's

gone through animal testing, phase one, phase two, and anywhere from phase two onwards. It's not always legitimate, but it's reasonable from that point on that it be part of clinical practice. So that would be my view of evidence. (Medical oncologist)

There was a tension in these specialists' accounts between the superiority of evidence (study design) and the superiority of result (individual patient outcomes). The biomedical hierarchy of evidence directly informed, *in theory*, what was perceived by the specialists as actual 'proof' of effectiveness. Randomised difference, in particular, was a constant delineating factor between those studies that could be used and those that could not. However, in practice, consultants were faced with the emotional and intuitive nature of advice giving and decision-making about best treatment:

Interviewer: At a practical level, what is evidence?
Clinician: Good evidence involves some randomised difference.
Interviewer: So [what about] a before-and-after study or a retrospective cohort study?
Clinician: I tend not to believe them particularly because empirical bias is so great because one: the cohorts always improve with time; the selection bias of the choice of patients is so gross, most of those turn out to be non-real differences ...
Interviewer: You won't have randomised for [some of your conditions]?
Clinician: Well, you sometimes do but they're a mish-mash of diseases, of like-diseases, and so it's very hard to tease some of it out. And then you get the value judgements you know all these sort of family issues, emotive issues that sort of push you into [trying a treatment] with poor evidence when you know it won't really work. (Medical oncologist)

Another respondent:
Clinician: We end up treating a lot of patients on pretty low-levels of evidence. So ... you know, we're treating quite a lot of patients on case-series basically without even ... I think we try not to treat too many on case reports but there are quite a few we treat on case series. But again, where there's potentially a reason for the treatment to have worked in the first place. So I think, if there is a randomised trial or ideally multiple randomised trials then that's where we feel most comfortable. But there's not many of our diseases that we get that for. (Haematological oncologist)

Another respondent:
Clinician: I guess [evidence-based medicine] is taking the best level of evidence and then applying it to that individual patient. At the

> patient level, there's always a degree of finesse about what you
> then do if there's a number of options available ... [in this
> hospital] I think we're reasonably evidence-based ... but there's a
> lot of parts of our practice ... where we probably do all kinds of
> things that are based on no evidence at all. (Haematological
> oncologist)

Whilst 'randomised difference' and 'survival advantage' were deployed
rhetorically in the interviews to delineate between studies that were appropriate
to guide clinical practice and those that were not, the emotive and subjective
nature (or art) of oncology consistently emerged in the respondents' talk around
evidence. Whilst study designs that were quasi-experimental (for example
before-and-after studies or non-randomised controlled trails) or observational
(for example cohort, incidence or case control studies) were viewed as 'biased'
and not actually constituting evidence *per se*, in contexts whereby options were
limited, such studies were viewed as 'appropriate' to inform decision-making
(albeit differentially according to specialty as shown below). Moreover, there
was awareness of the flaws of randomised difference, given that such studies can
include a range of conditions, stages of disease or aggressiveness, making such
evidence difficult to apply to an individual patient. As such in practice, and as seen
below, evidence was viewed considerably more broadly.

For example, whilst standard treatments for the most common malignancies
(for example adjunct chemotherapy for breast cancer) were based on 'high-level'
meta-analyses, many other oncological conditions required more subjective
judgement on the part of the consultants. In such contexts, the biomedical
hierarchy of evidence (Broom and Tovey 2007) was given little attention and
consultants worked with the limited data they had. Intuition was used to actively
gauge whether the treatment 'made sense' and fitted with their understandings of
general physiological and therapeutic effect. Such subjectivities provided some
justification for using a case study or case series to justify a treatment decision.

However, intuition and subjective judgement were in turn viewed as situated
within organisational cultures. Organisational practices shaped whether the
consultants-in-training were expected to be aware of the specific 'level of evidence'
and how cure rates were represented to patients. Moreover, there was a distinct
pattern of hierarchical delineation in terms of knowledge of evidence.

Intra-Professional and Inter-Organisational Differentiation

Inter-specialty differentiation in perspectives on evidence and indeed the
willingness to utilise particular forms of evidence to justify treatment decisions,
emerged as key themes in the interviews. Haematology was viewed (by *both*
the medical oncology and the haematology consultants) as being prepared to
regularly use 'inferior' forms of evidence (that is, case studies and case series)

to treat patients. In contrast, medical oncologists (again, from the perspectives of both specialist groups) were considered more conservative in terms of only utilising 'high-level' evidence. This difference – and the dialogue surrounding this issue within the interviews – was based on an inter-specialty debate regarding curability. Haematologists, from the perspective of the medical oncologists, justified the application of 'low' levels of evidence based on an historical and social expectation of cure for haematological malignancies; a fact promoted by the haematologists interviewed and disputed by the medical oncologists:

Clinician: Haematologists have a greater expectation of themselves to treat and cure their patients and are prepared to accept the lower level of evidence to try and achieve that …

Interviewer: What's the basis of that do you think?

Clinician: Well, I think there's just a different philosophy. Haematology evolved to have different ways of viewing [patient care]. I mean, most medical oncologists also view themselves as palliative care physicians and are fairly accepting of the fact that a lot of our patients won't do very well and take that into consideration. Whereas haematology, I think, just has a different philosophy in that you try and cure, prolong life … which is a good philosophy, but I think that means that patients are … over-treated. (Medical oncologist)

Another respondent:

Clinician: I think it is that [haematology] is more curable and the oncologist in the appropriate setting are probably as aggressive or more aggressive in some situations so I think it's just the nature of the disease. Probably because we are blasting away all the time, we're a bit more aggressive in general, but I think most of it is to do with the disease and the fact that diseases need that sort of approach. (Haematological oncologist)

Another respondent:

Clinician: Some [haematological malignancies] are more curable … yes. They [haematological consultants] focus on the ones that are. If you look at leukaemia, in general, in adults, some subsets will do well. You get cure-rates of 60 to 70 per cent. But the average cure rate is about 20 per cent which is pretty high-risk really. Large cell lymphoma you might pick up to the 60 to 70 per cent which is pretty good, but all the others are never curable and they die of it. (Medical oncologist, head of cancer services)

Discourses of curability and histories of success emerged as crucial in determining the quality of evidence acceptable for the individual specialty and specialist.

Individual successes within haematology, such as child leukaemia or large cell lymphoma, were seen to inflate the curative potential of haematological oncology and justify the application of 'inferior' evidence. Whereas in medical oncology, where the chances (and level of evidence) for cure may be the same, treatment would not go ahead. The relationship and involvement of medical oncology as a specialty in palliative care was viewed as crucial in shaping the tendency of medical oncologists to only treat when 'success' is likely and evidence is 'good'. The professional trajectory of haematology as 'experimental' (i.e. stem cell transplants) and 'curative' (i.e. child leukaemia or large cell lymphoma) was perceived as critical in driving the acceptability of low levels of evidence informing clinical practice.

It was clear from these clinicians' accounts that, whilst internal differences exist, oncology as a broad area of medicine is rather unique in terms of the seriousness of the conditions being treated. As such, in comparison to a surgical procedure in obstetrics (Pope 2003), or the treatment of depression in primary care (Armstrong 2002), there is a greater emphasis on the need to 'try something' and find the best evidence and 'run with it'. Thus, whilst the need for concrete evidence to rationalise toxicity was omnipresent, the need to treat in contexts of potential terminality often superseded this.

Managerialism, *res ipsa loquitur* and Deskilling in Oncology

Whilst intuition and judging effectiveness in terms of 'what is in front of you' emerged as crucial for some consultants and indeed a number of nurses (see discussion below), the senior consultants occupying quasi-managerial positions expressed considerable concern that consultants in their wards were making subjective judgements based upon individual patient response:

> Clinician: In clinical care ... you make a judgement call, and the trouble is, in my life, you've seen people go through various diseases on various treatments – I think melanoma being one of the best examples. It [melanoma] goes through cyclical things. People say, 'this is the best treatment'. Fabulous, it does this. And every time it goes into a randomised trial it's nothing because of selection bias. ... And, if you go on what you see in front of you, you think of all sorts of things. (Medical oncologist, head of cancer services)

Another respondent:

> Clinician: We should not be making decisions based on what is in front of us. This is a flaw in our organisational culture. The whole premise of EBM is going by evidence not what is in front of you. (Medical oncologist, head of haematology)

Thus, what emerged was a concern, in the context of a policy of EBM, around the potential for clinicians to 'miss the big picture' and provide treatment on the basis of biased results. Systematisation and increased managerialism were viewed, at least by some of the senior consultants interviewed, as providing a means of limiting such intuitive-based and anecdotal judgements. However, attempts at systematising clinical practice were also perceived to have adverse effects for many clinicians and therefore potentially for patient care.

The practicalities of applying the basic tenets of EBM were seen to necessarily involve some degree of systematisation (organisational or national clinical practice guidelines), however, a side-product of such processes was a perceived deskilling; particularly of advanced trainees or junior consultants who had limited knowledge of the particularities of the data they were drawing on. The use of information systems and organisational policies regarding best evidence for particular conditions were viewed as, at least in some cases, reducing the competency of doctors by taking away the need for awareness of the epistemological basis of the statistical probabilities being used (i.e. how was this figure produced, by whom, for which patients and in which contexts). The governmental and organisational pushes for EBM were seen as removing the need for doctors to 'know' the nature of statistical probabilities, and thus removing a critical element of professional identity and clinical judgement:

> Clinician: There's probably different answers [in terms of evidence and best treatment] depending on where people have trained and how sort of the units are structured. So, for our unit, there are a range of different therapy choices for any defined malignancy which have advantages and disadvantages for any individual depending upon their age. There are other units [in this city] that have, in general, a defined treatment or one treatment for any condition – so they fit the patient into the treatment. You [doctors in the other hospital cancer unit] know your unit protocol for cancer and they don't need to know the pros and cons of the data because that's the only one they use. Whereas in reality, we shouldn't be practicing like that. In reality, you should know the knowledge or the literature. ... The way they do it is bad for patient care and for doctors. (Haematological oncologist)

Another respondent:
> Clinician: As we get pushed for time and data-bases are set up we have less idea of the data we are communicating to patients. Sometimes you only know the statistic and have no idea of the actual studies backing it up. (Medical oncologist)

Another respondent:
> Clinician: I mean, sometimes, we tell patients figures that are based on our knowledge of what we've heard other doctors tell people; so

> without potentially knowing the exact details of the trials that they
> came from ... a lot of the particularly early advanced training years
> is pretty much repeating what you've heard your consultant say.
> But then as you get along, hopefully you interpret the data yourself
> ... certainly advance trainees coming into the system now know less
> that what we did. (Medical oncologist)

A process of organisationally-specific, managed deskilling was evident in some of these specialists' accounts whereby doctors were increasingly removed from the actual studies informing clinical decision-making (such as the trial designs used, publication types and country published). The need for increased systematisation of treatment processes was, in many cases, viewed as having negative influences on the ability of consultants (and advanced trainees) to *engage* with the trial data that informs treatment decision-making. What was interesting was the different attitudes towards advanced trainees, with one of the recruitment sites promoting critical decision making with multiple treatment options (trying to encourage clinical autonomy and individualism in their more junior doctors), whilst the other organisation systematised decision-making resulting in a perceived deskilling of the advanced trainees and eventually consultants. Such trajectories were based largely on the subjective interpretations of the senior consultants in terms of 'quality medicine', and were competitive in nature ('here we produce highly skilled and critical consultants' or 'here we have consistency in the care provided').

These findings resonate with Chapter 2 and the broader work of Timmermans and Angell (2001), specifically, the potential interplay between EBM and uncertainty in medical work. Whilst EBM may indeed flatten distinctions and inconsistencies in individual practice, it also evades the nuances and uncertainties important for training junior doctors in judgement and critical thinking. Developing the 'expert eye' is thus replaced with reliance on an 'expert system', changing the locus of control and potentially reducing the skill base of doctors in training.

Evidence-Based Nursing: Practices of Distinction and Distinction in Practice

A number of important themes emerged from our nurse interviews. Firstly, what constitutes evidence from a nursing perspective and how this relates to EBNP, and secondly, how such notions may deviate from conceptions of EBM within the medical community. What emerged in the nurses' accounts was a dialectical tension between the need for a nursing trajectory toward EBP while also advocating a grassroots resistance to a purely biomedical lens on what constitutes therapeutic legitimacy. As such, the interviewees talked both about evidence-based trajectories alongside practices of resistance and differentiation from medicine:

> Nurse: Evidence is stuff that is generated from your systematic collection of
>   research. But, it's also very much around how you're interpreting the

context of what is going on and how you use that in the moment with the patient. All this sort of stuff around their [the patients'] situation because that's all evidence as well that you use to interpret how to respond to different situations. (Oncology, academic/research role)

Another respondent:

Nurse: Evidence is probably, in some situations, can help you demonstrate effectiveness but effectiveness is much broader than what research can tell you. There is a lot of stuff that works because it works and we're never going to have really gold standard studies to tell us that. (Oncology, senior nurse)

Another respondent:

Nurse: Evidence-based nursing [is] based on the same principles as evidence-based medicine ... [but] we struggle to sort of acknowledge that forms of evidence come in many different types and we struggle with nurses' qualitative research as well being accepted [as evidence] and we still struggle in terms of using that [qualitative research] to guide practice. So it is different. Evidence-based nursing is probably more accepting of qualitative evidence in how it defines nursing. But nonetheless it's sort of, like, still the gold standard. It's still considered to be your randomised trials, so, in that sense, it's not different. (Oncology, academic/research role)

The nurse interviews illustrated considerable tension within nursing (at least from the perspectives of these interviewees) between a professional discourse of EBNP (i.e. the espousal, albeit indirectly, of the biomedical gold standard) and the principle and values that are seen to feed into the professional distinctiveness and legitimacy of nursing practice (Tovey and Adams 2003). Qualitative research was viewed as a key contribution of nursing researchers to healthcare knowledge production, and this was difficult to reconcile with a broader trajectory toward EBNP, which was perceived as aligned with the biomedical hierarchy of evidence (Broom and Tovey 2007). Thus, whilst EBNP was considered key to the overall professionalisation of nursing, restrictive notions of evidence were in turn viewed as delimiting the progress of nursing knowledge and practice. The subjectivity of patient care and the importance of maintaining a 'holistic approach' were constantly deployed rhetorically by these nurses to reinforce the key tenets of nursing practice. This is juxtaposed with the need to 'keep up with' the biomedical trajectory toward the systematisation and EBP. This conflict was often conceptualised as a tension between the need for legitimacy within a scientific model of medicine and a need for an articulation of the core of nursing (that is holism, spirituality, subjectivity, patient-centredness and patient advocacy).

The relationship of nursing to conceptions of evidence and discourses of EBM emerged as very much about the need for professional distinction from and alignment with medicine. Thus, whilst there is an academic trajectory toward retaining the 'traditional' values of the nursing role, a professionalising process of promoting a biomedicalised EBNP also emerges:

> Nurse:	Nursing has gone through that sort of phase of really defining its contribution to patient experience and patient outcomes. It has come to understand that through good research and systematic qualitative research exactly what it is that actually makes a difference to patients. So I mean, I think it was part of that professional stuff of the professionalising of nursing to see what its unique contribution to patient care is ... [nurses] don't think in the same way as in medicine. I think in medicine it's really quite black and white. Whereas much more so in nursing it is a continuum ... I think that, again, it comes back to that sort of base that I think it always has been based upon a holistic sort of model. (Oncology, academic/research role)

Another respondent:

> Nurse:	I think it's important to recognise that evidence-based practice is simply part of a world view we've been kind of aiming at ... but how do you measure things that are qualitative ...? We're talking about qualitative, holistic aspects of human beings that you can't measure and that's one of the problems of the evidence ... holism to me is the person being a whole being; not just a physical body, not just a physical body with a mind or a soul or a social life or whatever but a whole person integrated with spirit. (Oncology, academic/research role)

Meanwhile, there also emerged a supplementary tension between wider academic nursing agendas, the realities of clinical practice and multidisciplinary teams which involve active and delimiting hierarchies. Whilst elements within nursing in 'theory' may resist the biomedical hierarchy of evidence and the biomedical gold standard (espousing traditional nursing values including 'holism', interpretive epistemologies and 'patient-centred care') in practice, it would seem, nurses may find such a stance problematic:

> Nurse:	This is where some of this comes out; so, you've got academic nursing which very much wants to distinguish itself. But at the practice level they very much want to be part of that high-function medical team. The sort of research questions that I may be asked to look at are medical research, there's not a nursing ... thing in there ... anywhere you've got a medico, any acute care hospital, you've got a really, really strong medical dominance and I haven't seen that change in 30 years of working in hospitals. (Director of nursing research)

Another respondent:

Nurse: Where it's very process driven, so anything they get [taught outside the biomedical model] will soon be lost because, as we're saying, the nurses have to be work ready. What we mean by that is, they have to be able to get in and function and so they don't have to think about it. [Nurses trying to understand] evidence would actually throw out production within the hospital setting, so it probably wouldn't be included [in the curriculum]. (Oncology, academic/research role)

Another respondent:

Nurse: I guess evidence-based practice is … [long pause]. Well, I haven't seen a huge amount of it. As a nurse working in the hospital, there could be research about it, but nothing's provided to us about it. I haven't seen anyone too against it, but I guess I actually haven't seen much of it. (Oncology, junior)

What we see here is the way in which professional identity work and grassroots nursing practice diverge, with a desire to distinguish one's professional role but structural and organisational hierarchies that make achieving this delineation problematic. In order to ensure survival in a stretched Australian healthcare system, nurses, according to a number of the senior nurses interviewed here, need to be 'work ready' when they graduate (meaning, in this context, having 'practical skills' to work in a biomedically-oriented multidisciplinary team). Issues of distinction are thus potentially superseded by the need to survive in a context whereby much of the theoretical core of nursing identity is sidelined to support a biomedically-centred oncology service.

Just as resistance to EBNP was evident in the accounts of these nurses, imposing evidence-based guidelines to direct nursing practice also presented numerous difficulties:

Interviewer: Is there a difference between evidence-based practice in nursing and medicine?

Nurse: I think it's more evolved in medicine. … There's a lot of rhetoric in medicine around evidence-based medical practice but medical practice is very much individually-driven. So, consultants are trained to be autonomous in their decision-making. And there's a lot of rhetoric that will support standardisation of care in principle, but when it comes down to the individual [doctor], there's a conflict that becomes very clear, very quickly, around the autonomy of the decision-making and the principles around the standardisation of care which is based on evidence. Nurses' evidence-based practice is less-evolved … they're not actually trained to be autonomous decision-makers in the same context. So they tend to work as team-members.

Interviewer: So, are you suggesting that applying evidence is actually easier?

Nurse: Applying evidence is actually much, much more difficult because you have to actually breach cultural norms to make it part of that normal part of practice. (Director of cancer nursing).

Emerging from the interviews was a view of oncology nurses as developing more group-based, consensus-driven approaches to clinical practice that were not necessarily easy to shift. With nursing practices immersed in organisational culture, clinical practice can be very difficult to change regardless of the evidence available. Thus, although the consultants were largely individually driven and at times anti-consensus, a common view expressed was that it remained easier to prompt a change in practice due to new evidence in the medical environment when compared to nursing.

Discussion

This chapter has examined the ways in which a range of differently-positioned oncology consultants and nurses engage with notions of evidence and evidence-based medicine in clinical practice. An important feature of the accounts presented here was the differences between haematology and medical oncology in terms of the use of evidence and engagement with EBM. Specifically, the enactment of EBM emerged as situated within the speciality examined, with individual judgement and 'poor' evidence (such as case studies or case series) deemed much more acceptable within haematology than within medical oncology despite their broad similarities in overall cure rates and survival. The historicity and myth-making surrounding haematology as a 'harsh', 'experimental' and 'curative' speciality seemed critical in shaping the acceptability of clinicians' actions and the sub-cultural mediation of EBM. There also emerged broader idiosyncrasies in terms of the nature of oncological work and the need to abide by an EBM framework in everyday clinical decision-making. Whilst Pope (2003) identifies notions of the doing of surgery and Armstrong (2002) the indeterminacy of primary care as key to the mediation (and rejection) of EBM, here we see the dual threats of terminality (the need to treat) and toxicity as key mediating factors. Specifically, the tendency of oncology more broadly to be a more 'experimental' and thus 'intuitive' form of medicine, and the potential threat posed by an EBM-inspired therapeutic rationality.

Whilst there have been arguments regarding EBM as a potential contributing factor in the broader proletarianisation of biomedicine (Barnett, Barnett and Kearns1998, McKinlay and Stoeckle 1988, Weiss and Fitzpatrick 1997), drawing from the results of this study we suggest the need for a more differentiated and nuanced theoretical position. It would seem that EBM is concurrently consolidating oncological expertise through enhanced therapeutic rationality and objectivity, but also, potentially reducing the skill-base and critical judgement of junior doctors.

The accounts presented here illustrate the emergence of a managerial culture (albeit organisationally specific) promoting an EBM model of care that removes the need for registrars and advanced trainees (consultants in training) to critically assess evidence. The increased prominence of EBM's expert systems (that is, epidemiology, clinical practice guidelines and information systems) was perceived by a significant proportion of the consultants interviewed as facilitating a managed 'deskilling' in oncology (Timmermans and Angell 2001).

However, and consistent with other recent analyses of internal status differences within professional groups (Timmermans and Angell 2001, Friedson 2001), the transcendence of therapeutic rationality over clinical judgement/autonomy was hotly contested, with several of the consultants in managerial positions supporting the imposition of constraint on individual action in their departments. Specifically, several of the senior consultants told of the dangers of idealising grassroots clinical judgement and individual autonomy, and the necessity of strict organisational policies requiring evidence-based practice and the systematisation of evidence. In such contexts EBM has the potential to produce a new form of 'elite' medical expertise whereby clinical practice in a given unit is decided by a few consultants occupying senior positions. Resonating with Timmermans and Berg's (1997) notion of local universality, the enactment of EBM may in fact involve the re-skilling of senior doctors to focus on establishing and enforcing local 'best practice' which may still be idiosyncratic (as shown in the differences between the departments examined here) whilst still fitting into the EBM trajectory toward the systematisation of care. As seen in several of the accounts given here, this becomes problematic when the systematisation of care delimits the development of the 'expert eye' through debate and interaction between doctors regarding the nexus between abstract knowledge and clinical practice (Atkinson 1995).

A key rationale for imposing an EBM model was the danger of consultants' taking clinical outcomes 'at face value'. EBM, for several of the senior consultants, was to some extent seen as removing individual clinician bias/fallibility and improving overall outcomes for patients. Its clinical and technological manifestations were viewed as allowing oncologists to see the 'big picture' rather than being limited by their subjective interpretations of effectiveness and efficacy.

What emerged from this study is a contradictory view of EBM as experienced by differently positioned clinicians in specific oncology contexts. On the one hand, and as Goldenberg (2006: 2630) has argued, it actually reinforces the objective and detached status of oncology, further bolstering key aspects of the biomedical model. Furthermore, by ignoring the subjectivities and value judgements evident in knowledge production, it further obscures the connections between power and knowledge (Goldenberg 2006). However, the character of oncology (terminality and the pressure to treat) and the existence of organisationally-specific strategies of best practice (systematisation versus the promotion of critical thinking) mean that its impacts are situated and thus differentiated between organisations. As such, in the Australian context, and if the results presented here are reflected in other locations, we see the emergence of different (and competing) models of organisational structure, each presenting itself as practicing a superior form of oncology.

Whilst the doctors' interviews recounted the tensions between therapeutic rationality and subjectivity/individuality, the nurses' accounts drew out a complex dialectic between the need for biomedical, science-based legitimacy and a need to retain the values, goals and thus professional identity of nursing. The nurses represented nursing (and EBNP) as distinct, separate and broader than medicine and EBM. Qualitative research was drawn on as a key source of delineation, reflecting key epistemological divergences (patient narratives as legitimate knowledge) and ontological divergences (disease is subjective and experiential) from medicine. The nurse identity as 'holistic practitioner' was viewed as incorporating the emotional, cultural, spiritual and physiological spheres of patients care, and thus, EBNP also incorporated such values. However, while rhetorical distinctions regarding the different positioning of nursing in relation to evidence were consistent across the interviewees' accounts, there was clear recognition that these were often difficult to actualise in everyday nursing work. Distinctions between the specialties in nursing in this context are not clear; what is clear is the potential for EBM to both validate and problematise nursing philosophy and practice; much like in medicine.

Much work is needed to explore the experiences of oncologists in terms of the tensions between professional identity, organisational culture and individual judgement; the study reported here merely sought to begin this process with a select group of clinicians in the specific context of Australian cancer care. The focus for sociologists should now be on how other sites of clinical work (and patient care) are changing under the rubric of EBM; identifying key sites of resistance to, or translation of, EBM; and, the character of inter- and intra-specialty differentiation. This book is a significant step in the right direction in terms of revealing the cultures of knowledge work and evidence utilisation. It is only then that we will fully understand how EBHC as a contemporary social movement is shaping the nature of medical work and patient care.

Acknowledgements

We thank the clinicians for the willingness to commit their valuable time to this project. Parts of this chapter were originally published in 2009 in the journal *Social Science and Medicine*, 68(1), 192–200.

References

Armstrong, D. 2002. Clinical autonomy, individual and collective. *Social Science and Medicine*, 55(10), 1771–7.
Atkinson, P. 1995. *Medical Talk and Medical Work*. Thousand Oaks: Sage.

Barnett, R., Barnett, P. and Kearns, R. 1998. Declining professional dominance? Trends in the proletarianisation of primary care in New Zealand. *Social Science and Medicine*, 46(2), 193–207.

Boschma, G. 1994. The meaning of holism in nursing: Historical shifts in holistic nursing ideas. *Public Health Nursing*, 11(5), 324–30.

Broom, A. and Tovey, P. 2007. Therapeutic pluralism? Evidence, power and legitimacy in UK cancer services. *Sociology of Health and Illness*, 29(3), 551–69.

Chabner, B. and Roberts, T. 2005. Chemotherapy and the war on cancer. *Nature Reviews Cancer*, 5, 65–72.

Cox, J. 2000. Evidence in oncology: The Janeway lecture. *Cancer Journal*, 6(6), 351–7.

Davidson, N. 2007. The maturation of medical oncology. *The Lancet Oncology*, 8(6), 457–8.

De Vries, R. and Lemmens, T. 2006. The social and cultural shaping and medical evidence. *Social Science and Medicine*, 62(11), 2694–706.

Goldenberg, M. 2006. On evidence and evidence-based medicine: Lessons from the philosophy of science. *Social Science and Medicine*, 62(11), 2621–32.

Greenhalgh, T. 1999. Narrative based medicine in an evidence based world. *British Medical Journal*, 318, 323–5.

Helms, J. 2006. Complementary and alternative therapies: A new frontier for nursing education? *Journal of Nursing Education*, 45(3), 117–23.

Ioannidis, J., Schmid, C. and Lau, J. 2000. Meta-analysis in hematology and oncology. *Hematology/Oncology Clinics of North America*, 14(4), 973–91.

Kessenich, C., Guyatt, G. and DiCenso, A. 1997. Teaching nursing students evidence-based nursing. *Nurse Educator*, 22(6), 25–9.

Lambert, H. 2006. Accounting for EBM: Notions of evidence in medicine. *Social Science and Medicine*, 62(11), 2633–45.

Light, K. 1997. Florence Nightingale and holistic philosophy. *Journal of Holistic Nursing*, 15(1), 25–40.

McKinlay, J. and Stoeckle, J. 1988. Corporatisation and the social transformation of doctoring. *International Journal of Health Services*, 18(2), 191–205.

Pope, C. 2003. Resisting evidence: The study of evidence-based medicine as a contemporary social movement. *Health*, 7(3), 267–82.

Timmermans, S. and Angell, A. 2001. Evidence-based medicine, clinical uncertainty, and learning to doctor. *Journal of Health and Social Behavior*, 42(4), 342–59.

Timmermans, S. and Berg, M. 1997. Standardization in action: Achieving local universality through medical protocols. *Social Studies of Science*, 27(2), 273–305.

Tovey, P. and Adams, J. 2003. Nostalgic and nostophobic referencing and the authentication of nurses' use of complementary therapies. *Social Science and Medicine*, 56(7), 1469–80.

Tredaniel, J., Blay, J., Goldwasser, F., Asselain, B., Koscielny, S., de Labareyre, C., Balogh, N., Bismut, H., Misset, J. and Marty M. 2005. Decision making process in oncology practice. *Critical Reviews in Oncology-Hematology*, 54(3), 165–70.

Weiss, M. and Fitzpatrick, R. 1997. Challenges to medicine: The case of prescribing. *Sociology of Health and Illness*, 19(3), 297–327.

PART III
Evidence on the Margins

Chapter 7

Evidence-Based Health Care and Complementary and Alternative Medicine

Kevin Dew

Introduction

At the heart of the issue of what constitutes acceptable therapeutic practice is the question of what therapeutic practice should be based on. The ideal propounded by many in the medical profession is that scientific research is the basis of practice; invalid therapies are those that are scientifically untested, a criticism levelled at complementary and alternative medicine (CAM). Moreover, this ideal propounds that a practitioner must be suitably trained at a reputable scientific institution where training is based on the most up-to-date scientific research (Bosk 1986, Rosenthal 1995). Once trained, practitioners should keep up with developments in their field with mechanisms put in place to ensure this occurs. A number of problems arise if this view is held. Much of what medical practitioners do, like CAM, has not been subjected to rigorous scientific scrutiny. The uncertainties of medical practice (Wallis 2009) and research (Henry 2006), variability amongst practitioners (Eddy 1984), and the untested basis of much of medical practice (Smith 1991) have been well documented. Even where there is evidence that is regarded as authoritative by evidence-based medical standards, where interventions have been successfully tested using randomised controlled trials (RCTs), there is still the problem of applying it to 'the specific circumstances of an individual patient' (Klein, Day and Redmayne 1996: 92).

Medical professionals react to the uncertainty of medical practice in different ways. One prominent response has been the development of evidence-based medicine (EBM), which promotes a hierarchy of authority. EBM developed in an effort to orient medicine towards what was perceived as the existing science and knowledge base. It became increasingly important in the 1990s, although Lohr and colleagues suggest that a landmark treatise was Archie Cochrane's 1972 text *Effectiveness and Efficacy* (Lohr, Eleazer and Mauskopf 1998). At the top of the EBM hierarchy of evidence for interventions is the RCT while the bottom level is where guidelines are based on the consensus of experts. In a Weberian sense this exhibits a gradient from authority based on a narrow notion of rational science to a traditional authority (Weber 1948).

Getting the Evidence

A number of problems have been identified with basing clinical practice on EBM. Firstly, patient selection for many RCTs has tended to be biased with middle aged white males who have no co-existing conditions constituting a significant proportion of the researched population (Lohr, Eleazer and Mauskopf 1998). In a clinical setting, physicians are faced with a patient population that is far more diverse. Thus, the application of EBM in practice is problematic, highlighting the impact of a difference between efficacy and effectiveness. Efficacy 'requires that a clinical procedure achieves benefits to individuals in defined populations (often defined narrowly) when it is applied under ideal or optimal circumstances' (Lohr, Eleazer and Mauskopf 1998: 8). Effectiveness applies to the clinical setting where a procedure should do more harm than good. It has been shown that many interventions found by RCT to be efficacious do not lead to improved outcomes when translated into practice (Glasgow, Vogt and Boles 1999). This is exacerbated by the increasing tendency of commercial companies to conduct RCTs for pharmaceuticals in what are termed non-traditional research locations such as Latin America and Eastern Europe (Petryna 2007). Petryna (2007: 24) reports a scientific advisor of a contract research organisation stating that: 'companies can now pick and choose populations in order to get a most pronounced drug benefit signal as well as a "no-harm" signal'. This effect may be achieved through trial recruitment strategies which, for example, can recruit from treatment-naive groups who have very little history of pharmaceutical use even though the results are generalized to treatment-saturated markets with many people on multiple medications (Petryna 2007). As such, the evidence for EBM, particularly pharmaceuticals, has significant limitations.

EBM and CAM can come into conflict over evidentiary claims. Biomedicine emphasises explanations based in the biological and chemical sciences and, as has been stated, the primacy of the RCT. In contrast, the evidence base for many CAM practices is based on canonical texts and extensive clinical experience (Polich, Dole and Kaptchuk 2010). Although advocates of EBM argue that decisions should be based on the most appropriate evidence, therefore potentially extending beyond RCTs in the context of interventions, RCTs still dominate systematic reviews aimed at influencing treatment decision-making (Green 2000). However, as EBM interventions place an emphasis on outcomes rather than explanations this has some potential advantages for CAM (Willis and White 2004). If a CAM treatment is found to work, for example homeopathy, then it should not matter that the mechanisms of the therapy's action make no sense to biomedicine in biological or chemical terms. EBM could, paradoxically, provide an evidentiary base that undermines the claims of biomedicine. There are, however, some important constraints on that potential.

One limitation is that researchers studying CAM confront a number of barriers that researchers studying orthodox medicine do not. For example, instead of reviewers of journals assessing the science behind the treatment, their review comments have been known to simply disparage the CAM therapy with statements such as 'acupuncture is a bunch of crap' (Polich, Dole and Kaptchuk 2010: 114). This sort of response was reported by Polich and colleagues who interviewed CAM researchers who were principal investigators on projects funded by the National Institutes of Health's National Center for Complementary and Alternative Medicine in the USA. These emotive reactions from reviewers of their research have made it more difficult for CAM research articles to be published in comparison to those based on orthodox research. This bias against CAM research is further compounded by the kinds of standardisation required for RCT type studies. Some CAM researchers acknowledge that standardising protocols do not conform to CAM approaches because treatments are supposed to be unique to each individual (Polich, Dole and Kaptchuk 2010). Thus, it is difficult for CAM researchers to build up an evidence-base for CAM practitioners both because their research is subject to discrimination by reviewers and because standardisation requirements can be contradictory to CAM practice.

It can be noted that there are a range of therapeutic validations. Therapies may be scientifically tested and orthodox, untested and orthodox, tested and unorthodox or untested and unorthodox. To divide medical practice into orthodox and unorthodox or mainstream and alternative categories is a gross simplification of a very complex situation. The boundary between CAM and orthodox medicine is not clear cut, and what gets labelled alternative at any particular time is dependent upon prevailing medical ideologies, cultural norms and the social organisation and political power of the medical profession and other health practitioners (Dew 2001). Furthermore, what counts as evidence is variable, at various times and for different groups it can be empirical observations, theoretical foundations or experiential understandings (see, for example, Atkinson 1997, Foucault 2003, Nutton 2006, R. Porter 2006). However, the valorisation of EBM with its particular form of empiricism does, theoretically at least, put pressure on those using CAM approaches to establish the legitimacy of their therapy at this sociohistorical juncture.

The Biopsychosocial and the Biomedical

Not only does EBM place pressure on CAM practitioners to provide a legitimised evidential base, but an unintended consequence of the EBM movement is that it can act as a mechanism to steer medical practitioners away from biomedicine. Since the 1950s there has been a movement within the medical profession towards biopsychosocial medicine in contrast to a more limited biomedical model (Checkland et al. 2008). Variations on this theme have included patient-centred medicine and holistic medicine, which have been focused around general practice. This has been described by David Armstrong as an attempt by primary care physicians to redefine themselves in order to find a viable position within the medical marketplace (Armstrong 1982). Armstrong (1982: 119) argues that in this type of model 'the whole person is a multidimensional rather than a unitary being'. This anti-reductionist view became incorporated in publications by the Royal College of General Practitioners in the 1970s where general practice was defined as concerning itself with 'the patient's total experience of illness' (Checkland et al. 2008: 790). The term biopsychosocial was coined in 1972, conceptualising disease as a manifestation of biological, psychological, social and cultural conditions (Checkland et al. 2008). However, this extension of medical practice beyond the biological and physical into the psychological and social runs counter to the movement of EBM. It is as hard to scientifically test counselling, a part of the therapeutic regimen of the biopsychosocial practitioner, as it is to test homoeopathy (Dew 2001). Therefore, if EBM does not provide the legitimacy, some other justification for utilising biopsychosocial and related approaches is required.

Legitimacy and the Art of Medicine

Linking EBM to forms of professional accountability restricts the art of medicine and the autonomy of the practitioner. Drawing on Weber, it has been argued that evidence-based practice undermines traditional clinical expertise as clinicians are increasingly required to point to an external evidentiary authority in order to provide justification for their decisions as opposed to relying on their own experience (Lipman 2000). In what has been termed scientific-bureaucratic medicine, bureaucracies oversee and control the implementation of evidence-based practice further undermining the clinical autonomy of practitioners (Checkland et al. 2008, Lipman 2000).

Contemporary legitimation developments in medical practices relate to what Anspach terms the ecology of knowledge, where interactive cues in assessing problems and intervening are devalued in relation to technological cues (Anspach 1987). That is, certain forms of knowing are considered not to provide sufficient warrant for the actions of diagnosis and intervention, whilst other forms of knowing do. A warrant for actions provides a publicly available form of accounting. Goodwin and Mort refer to the role of professional accountability practices in legitimising health care practices in the face of an unattainable ideal of certainty in relation to knowledge, diagnoses and practices (Goodwin and Mort 2010). For health professionals, professional governing bodies establish the standards by which members of the profession are held accountable. One has to be able to demonstrate that decisions and actions are defensible in relation to codes of conduct and other professional standards. Practitioners who do not conform to the standards of professional accountability need to provide a warrant for their non-conformity. As will be discussed, one particularly important warrant for their actions from GPs who use CAM relates to a narrative of crisis.

Codes of conduct and professional standards include following guidelines, protocols and practice policies, which according to Berg induce similar actions in that 'they can be read as a set of *instructions* telling medical personnel to do a certain thing in a certain situation' (Berg 1997: 2). Protocols can be termed procedural standards and these attempt to specify the processes by which diagnoses are made and treatment plans are determined and implemented (Timmermans and Berg 2003). These protocols relate to efforts to standardise medicine, and as such define medical practice as the logical and sequential application of science. The standardisation process is further reinforced as EBM constitutes a major element in quality assurance and medical audit (Lohr, Eleazer and Mauskopf 1998).

Standardisation is a way of dealing with huge variations in medical practice with widely varying outcomes. However, one possible consequence of the standardisation of medical practice is the limit it places on patient choice. The clinical agenda of a check-list protocol can supersede the patient's agenda (Collins et al. 1997, Rhodes et al. 2006). This should not be a pre-determined conclusion however, for as Timmermans and Berg point out, standardisation in clinical practice is itself a process of dynamic change, and in order to understand that change, attention needs to be given to how standardisation reorders practices (Timmermans and Berg 2003). It cannot be assumed that attempts to standardise medical practices through such means as requiring the use of protocols will have the intended outcome. Indeed, as has been demonstrated by detailed analysis of interactions between patients and clinicians, there are many means by which clinicians can ignore, undermine or utilize protocols and standardised procedures (Dew et al. 2005a, Dew et al. 2010).

To illustrate this in the context of CAM, the Medical Council of New Zealand's guidelines for medical practitioners who use CAM places the onus on the practitioners 'to inform the patient not only of the nature of the alternative treatment offered but also the extent to which that is consistent with conventional theories of medicine' (Medical Council of New Zealand 2005). Research on consultations has demonstrated that this attempt at a standardised approach for all practitioners is not easily executed as it requires the practitioner to understand the mechanisms by which CAM treatments work (Dew et al. 2008). There are documented instances where medical practitioners advise patients to try out particular supplements, for example Evening Primrose oil for premenstrual problems, but do not appear to have any specific information on how the supplement might work. The advice is empirically-based, where the practitioners suggest a trial-like approach of CAM to their patients. There is an absence of a discussion of the nature of the treatment, as required by guidelines, because the practitioner does not have the theoretical understanding to engage in such a discussion. This example shows how attempts at standardisation through guidelines do not necessarily align with the actual activities of practitioners.

Modernity and Clinical Legibility

One way of conceptualising the development of evidence-based medicine and the plethora of other phenomena that seek to standardise clinical practice is to consider them as part of a long historical process of simplification. James Scott argues that in high modernity we witness a process whereby what was once socially illegible or opaque is rendered legible and therefore administratively convenient. This process is achieved through rationalisation and standardisation. As examples of this, Scott refers to the ways in which surnames have been imposed on populations, maps drawn and weights and measures standardised across regions to promote statecraft in various forms – ensuring taxes can be collected, that trade can occur efficiently and that military power may be enhanced (Scott 1998).

This same process of rationalising and standardising for the purposes of statecraft can be witnessed in the clinical consultation. An extremely powerful standardisation apparatus in health care has been assembled over recent decades that combines, among other things, management systems that bring together computer technologies and the use of protocols, health economics and rationing, population health perspectives, a quantification rhetoric and a particular scientific hierarchy of authority for interventions (with RCTs at the top). Efforts over the last few decades have been made to overcome the diversity and variability of local clinical practices, to replace practical knowledge with formal systems. As such the means are set in place for more centralised control over clinical activities (Dew in press).

As Scott notes, there are problems with the imposition of standardisation on a messy reality: 'Designed or planned social order is necessarily schematic; it always ignores essential features of any real, functioning social order' (Scott 1998: 6). Practical knowledge and informal processes are necessary antidotes to simplification. We see in the response to rationing in clinical decision-making that practitioners develop their own informal systems to resist the implied linear processes (Dew et al. 2010). Thus, the straightforward imposition of a uniform order is elusive and the impacts of standardisation should not be overstated.

The work of Scott and others (see, for example, T. Porter 1995) suggests, in line with Weber, inexorable processes of standardisation and rationalisation occurring in society. Medical practice, like other aspects of social life, is being caught up in these processes. However, there are spaces of resistance. The following draws on research conducted with seven medical practitioners who were identified in relation to debates on legislation regulating the medical profession in New Zealand (Dew 2003). The medical practitioners practised a range of different therapies, including different forms of acupuncture, nutrition-focused and anthroposophical medicine, a spiritual and holistic approach to medicine developed by Rudolf Steiner. The focus of this chapter is how these medical practitioners who use CAM resist the apparatus of evidence-based models. These practitioners are a particularly interesting case as they, at some level, explicitly reject the medical paradigm of evidence and therefore draw on other evidential sources to support their therapeutic authority. There is no claim being made here that the views expressed by these practitioners are representative of medical practitioners who use CAM – but they do provide insight into forms of resistance in respect to the dominant biomedical narratives of evidence.

The Concept of Science

One way that these respondents defend a space for CAM in the face of EBM is to provide an expanded account of science. A respondent who used electro-acupuncture illustrates this:

> The scientific method involves basically observation, interpretation of the observations and putting the theory to these observations. Now we do that regardless of whether you have got lab tests, double-blind studies and all that other sort of stuff. ... The whole system of Chinese medicine is very scientific in that true sense, of observations, interpretations and so on. (Electro-acupuncturist)

This representative excerpt shows that practices rely on observations that are linked to theories. It is empirically grounded and therefore 'scientific in that true sense'. Thus, Chinese medicine was not only considered to be a science, but it in some sense a more pure or true form of science than 'lab tests, double-blind studies and all that other sort of stuff'.

Here is a claim to a truer science where theory is tested, but not in the format of an RCT. Exactly how theory is tested is not elaborated, but one could postulate that this is more like an experimental science than a randomised controlled trial, where practices are tried out and a positive reaction reinforces belief in that practice. Where the reaction is negative the practice is modified or abandoned. In this framework science is a process, not simply an outcome. This indeed reflects close observational work of clinical practice, where diagnoses are often a post hoc attribution in response to the results of some intervention (Goodwin and Mort 2010). Hypotheses are suggested, which are then empirically tested with a medication or a treatment, and depending upon the response the candidate diagnosis is supported or rejected.

A claim was made by some practitioners that their therapies were justified on the basis of a different sort of science, or an alternative science. This can be seen in the account provided by an anthroposophical doctor who referred to anthroposophy as spiritual science. He stated that:

> Anthroposophy – actually the name that Rudolph Steiner gave to it is spiritual science. And it is actually very scientific – it is at least as scientific as the rest of science. And you enlarge science to encompass things – with the same way [that] I can measure and work with a table or with glass or experiments, I can actually do that also with the so-called life forces. There are a lot of books – and chromatographic methods and bio-dynamic agriculture and electrophoresis tests, and blood sensitive crystallisation tests, where you can actually make these etheric forces visible. There are a lot of things that you can actually – what is not directly visible with your five senses you can use the same rigour of scientific investigation in those fields. And then you find the same reproducible results. And that is what I think is science. (Anthroposophical doctor)

Here the methods of science are valorised for their 'rigour', but the claim is made that this same rigour applies to this particular CAM approach – it is simply that the approach extends beyond the 'five senses'. Instead of invoking an EBM hierarchy this doctor draws up a different hierarchy. There is a form of legitimation that is based on 'a lot of books'. As such, this implies a body of knowledge that has been built up, in line with Polich's argument that CAM practitioners draw on particular canons or texts as sources of legitimacy (Polich, Dole and Kaptchuk 2010). The observations made do not appear from nowhere and are not based on an individual's idiosyncrasies. Rather, they are based on prior theoretical understandings and development. In addition, the therapeutic approach is based on something measurable and by technologies that have been specifically developed to undertake the measuring – to make visible that what is normally invisible. Just as a cardiologist can render visible the workings of the heart through electro-cardiograms, the anthroposophists can render visible etheric forces that influence wellbeing. Evidence is not rejected, science is not rejected, and a technological means of diagnosis is not rejected. But these are all positioned within a different view of the world.

The anthroposophical doctor suggested that medicine itself was not a science. This claim was not made in this way by other respondents and related to his views that science deals with categories while medicine deals with individuals; science with uniformity, medicine with difference; science with the object, medicine with the subject. This is perhaps the crucial point in identifying the different worldviews discussed here. These views do not constitute a rejection of science, but that a very tight boundary is placed around what science can say. Medicine draws on science but is not a science because it deals with unique individuals. Science from this perspective deals with categories and groups, and as such individual differences cannot be accounted for. Patients are to be subjected to standardised procedures that, in an ideal world, follow protocols based on evidence-based medicine. As such, science can have an impact on the practice of medicine, but is not the complete answer. Understandings that take into account the particular individual must be drawn on in order to complete science in relation to clinical practice.

The following is taken from an interview with a primary care medical practitioner who had voiced criticisms in the medical media of medical practitioners who used CAM. The following excerpt illustrates an orthodox narrative about evidence:

> But I am also a scientist and I believe that the western paradigm of science is what we know as truth. ... I think there is some science in acupuncture. ... But what I have read of just about every other fringe activity, and they go in a sort of Gaussian curve from the pretty scientific, with acupuncture down this end through homoeopathy down to iridology and colour therapy and all the real weirdoes down this end – shining different coloured lights in your eyes and so on. So there are scientific studies which show that those ones are useless, there seems to have been some scientific studies which show that these other ones are

pretty useful, and in the middle there you've got this huge bunch of believers that take it on almost like a religion. (Primary care practitioner)

In this excerpt the practitioner draws on the well known imagery of the Gaussian or bell curve. For this practitioner there is room for CAM practices in medical practice as long as they could be placed in the category of being 'pretty scientific' and not in the category of the 'useless'. This is not a simple either/or dichotomy about acceptable practices, as might be suggested from a notion of absolute proof of efficacy. Instead, there is a gradation where some approaches have different quantities of science associated with them. Implicit in this excerpt is an idea that science will tease out what works and what does not work, and in opposition to science is belief. Underpinning this is an epistemological position that beliefs and theories can be separated out through scientific observations and that science itself is a neutral and value-free arbiter of the one correct view of the world.

For this primary care practitioner an orthodox narrative of science breaks down to some extent in the complexities of primary care practice where the high technology tools and resources required for certainty in practice are not readily available. Here he discusses the issue of uncertainty in medical practice, and how he dealt with it:

> There is another commonly held belief which is that the general practitioner must live with uncertainty whereas the hospital doctor can be pretty sure of diagnoses, has all the tests immediately available, isn't so concerned about cost containment. ... But as general practitioners we very often can recognise that this patient hasn't got something that is progressive or terminal, or is unlikely to be, and so the saying is that we live with uncertainty because in many of our cases we never make a diagnosis. I was in general practice for 20 years and I think I always made a diagnosis. Now it might not have been a 100 per cent certain diagnosis, it might not have been expressed in pathological terms, but there was always a name for what the person had and I suppose it depends on how you define the word diagnosis. To me a diagnosis is a name that the patient and me agree to put to what is wrong. That is not in scientific terms. (Primary care practitioner)

There are many points we can take from this excerpt. One is an explicit rejection of science as the basis for the primary care practitioner's authority – 'that is not in scientific terms'. The diagnosis here is reached by a form of consensus between him and the patient – an expression perhaps of the concept of patient-centred medicine or concordance. Patient-centred medicine has been of interest in general practice since the 1970s (Mead and Bower 2000) and concordance approaches since the late 1990s. The latter has been defined as:

> An agreement reached after negotiation between a patient and a healthcare professional that respects the beliefs and wishes of the patient in determining

whether, when, and how medicines are to be taken. (Dickinson, Wilkie and Harris 1999: 787)

What is suggested by the primary care practitioner is something rather more than patient concordance. He suggests that the patient determines, in negotiation with the practitioner, what the diagnosis is with the treatment plan following diagnosis. That is, the hierarchy of EBM is explicitly rejected as a new non-EBM element is introduced as a source of evidence – the patient's views. This aligns with developments in general practice since at least the 1950s that have been discussed, where biomedicine was supplemented by a concern for the patient experience and patient choice (Checkland et al. 2008).

This practitioner also makes a contrast with the more technologically resourced practitioners in the hospital setting who have the advantage of not being so concerned with 'cost containment' and who can, because of access to those costly resources, be 'pretty sure of diagnoses'. Like the anthroposophical doctor this practitioner valorises what can be rendered visible through technology, but as the technologies available to him are limited he falls back on some other form of legitimation – an agreed upon diagnosis.

The same practitioner draws on different notions of clinical practice depending upon the context. If the context is other CAM practices, the requirement is to be scientific within an EBM framework. If the context is his practice, then 'scientific terms' can be rejected and a non-EBM framework of evidence may be called upon.

What these excerpts show is the flexibility of the concept of science as deployed by practitioners. In all cases a narrow definition of science is rejected in favour of an expanded version. The next section details the limited, but by no means unimportant, place of science for those practitioners who use CAM.

Biomedical Crises and CAM Solutions: Linking the Past to the Present

Accounts of why these medically trained doctors initially got interested in CAM approaches are revealing. There has been little research to date that explores the narratives of medical practitioners who started using CAM in their practice. These narratives show how practitioners found their medical training provided limited opportunities to respond to their patients in a way that enhanced patients' wellbeing. All the medical practitioners provide a narrative in which the limitations of biomedicine led to a crisis of sorts in their own practice that prompted them to search for solutions outside those learnt during medical education. The search led them away from an EBM framework because it did not work in the situations they faced nor did it provide them with the resources to practise in a way they believed they should.

A frequent feature of these narratives is the depiction of a continuity of the self with the past. Some of the narratives convey a self-description categorised in terms of a pre-medical training, medical and then post-medical training self.

The medical self gains science, but loses something that the pre-medical self had or desired. The post-medical self unites what was gained with what was lost; a narrative of loss and recovery. EBM and the scientific self are gained, but at a price that is too great. However, EBM and science are not rejected – something extra has now been added, something recovered from the past relating to their sense of identity and their understanding of what it is to be a healer.

The following is from a medical practitioner who had a particular focus on diet:

> I think if you go back, it is really your upbringing that makes a huge difference. You change a lot afterwards. I was brought up in war time in a country area where my father did all the gardening. And I look back, there were no sprays, no chemicals, no additives, no preservatives. There were problems, I mean who wants to go back to the early 1940s really? But the bringing up was pretty good. We had a lot of fresh air, we were outside, our water didn't have anything added to it. We had a good positive attitude for health. My grandmother was one of the sort of early days pioneer ladies. So I think that made a huge difference to how really our health was. We were breast fed and all the usual things that go with it. A mother who knew about home first-aid. (Nutritional practitioner)

In this excerpt there is a presentation of a pre-medical self that experienced a particular way of living. One could describe this narrative as one of naturalness, purity and self-sufficiency. The narrative then takes a turn:

> But then I went to medical school at Dunedin, and did my Houseman and Registrar years in Christchurch. And I think I came out of medical school just the way that probably most people do. You know, it was the time of the super antibiotics, cortisones, birth control pill. I thought, wow, we've got something for everybody, we are really smart people. And you know, it was quite an exciting time in ways. (Nutritional practitioner)

Here the benefits of biomedicine are clearly presented and the positive support this provided for the practitioner's identity: 'we are really smart people'. This not only affirms the knowledge-base of biomedicine but also the idea of biomedicine as a collective enterprise that all the medical students engaged in. The paradigm of science is characterised as a collective effort with medical practice reaping the rewards of technological and pharmaceutical advances and new understandings of the body. The narrative then takes a further turn:

> But then I went into general practice … and just gradually it sort of dawned on me the sort of problems of the things that we were holding on to. You know I am not giving away medicine, medicine is my background, there are lots of good things there. But there were lots of other problems with it. With the kinds of

pills we used, and dosages, and the people were different, and I presumed what people's diets were like, and stress and how it had an effect upon them.

And so gradually I suppose I changed ... there was a whole number of things that probably started me thinking again. And that is there was cancer in my husband's family, both his sisters died of cancer at 34, and his father died of cancer at the age of 51. I then had a friend who came to me who had done a PhD in paediatrics who sort of said 'what did I know about laetrile and diet and things for cancer', her mother had cancer and she was terribly upset. And I didn't really know anything about these things. (Nutritional practitioner)

The above interviewee recounts a growing concern about the limited nature of biomedicine in relation to people's lives, a theme articulated by others in the study. For her, individual variability in response to medications and issues related to diet and stress highlighted particular limits to biomedicine. This is followed by the development of a crisis – on the one hand cancer in the family and premature death which by implication biomedicine could do nothing about, and then a realisation of a limited knowledge base when asked by a colleague about laetrile. Laetrile is an extract from apricot seeds that has been used as an alternative treatment for cancer but has been widely criticised by many in the medical profession (Broom 2009b, Hess 1997). In this narrative there is a sense of helplessness in the face of fatal disease and a threat to identity due to a lack of knowledge about approaches to potentially fatal diseases. Such a crisis facilitates the search for alternatives to biomedicine, which for this respondent involves a return to the childhood experience of a healthy diet and lifestyle.

The following is from the anthroposophical doctor. In the earlier part of the narrative, not recorded below, the doctor refers to the importance of philosophy in his own childhood education in Europe. He then moves on to the following:

I was actually a promising young scientific doctor. Then I felt though that it seemed to me that you had, actually if you looked just a little bit further than just the symptoms, that you had certain people that were more or less predisposed to certain illnesses, and I felt that it was very interesting that it had something to do with a warm personality or a cold personality, and something like warm diseases, febrile illnesses and cold illnesses, more degenerative illness, and I was very intrigued but I didn't go any further.

We sent our child, our son, to the local school at the age five. I felt that coming from Holland where you started at seven we were actually very unhappy with that, so we took him out and looked for an alternative. There was none apart from the Rudolph Steiner School. We sent him there, and that was the first time when I actually heard about Anthroposophy at the Rudolph Steiner School.

Then I had a patient a few weeks later who had measles meningitis, it was a patient of 50, a very peculiar thing. And she had a lot of headache and a lot of pain and neck stiffness and there was nothing I could do because this was measles and measles you can't do anything. So she was on pethidine and things like that and I got really frustrated. I felt I am a doctor, I want to help the patient and I can't, because our axioma says there is nothing that you can do for a virus. (Anthroposophical doctor)

There are some striking similarities in the narrative of the anthroposophical doctor and that of the nutritional practitioner. In particular, both practitioners described a crisis of faith in biomedicine. The practitioner goes on:

I had heard about one doctor who did different ways of medicine, he was a retired doctor ... and I phoned him and I said doctor I have no idea what you work from but is there anything that I could do. And he said why don't you come along ... and I came there and he said, look, I work from Anthroposophy and that has something to do with Rudolph Steiner, and I said that is interesting I have just sent my son there to the school. (Anthroposophical doctor)

The school referred to is a Rudolph Steiner school that is based upon anthroposophical principles. The doctor who was contacted explained some of the principles of anthroposophical medicine:

[H]e said one of the polarities that we work with is the polarity of inflammation versus sclerosis, versus degenerative illnesses, because we feel that there are certain acute illness, hot illnesses, and cold ones. And I said, but that is exactly where my question was. So that really clicked. And then I worked with him a lot. ... Also standing with one foot firmly in conventional medicine because I want to be able to choose as a doctor what I think is best, and that may be an antibiotic, or it may be quartz D30 you know. (Anthroposophical doctor)

Similar to the earlier narratives, the practitioner ends by affirming that biomedicine is important, but indicating that he now has more. To paraphrase this, for these practitioners, the science of biomedicine is not enough and something else had to be added. Biomedicine is not able to provide answers in particular situations and the practitioners seek some other means of responding to those situations. They find a different way of responding to ill-health and disease from those taught to them in medical school.

The following excerpt is from an interview with the doctor who used electro-acupuncture. This respondent was Asian and in his narrative he does not specifically refer to his upbringing or any cultural concepts learnt as a child, but turns to an 'old Chinese doctor' when biomedicine does not work:

My interest first of all started by the fact that when I was in Auckland, after coming back from overseas with my postgraduate training in anaesthetics, that I suffered from hay fever ... one year I had it very bad, and I tried all sorts of nasal spray, anti-histamines, whatever there was in the pharmacopoeia I sort of tried and it was not working. More or less out of desperation I contacted an old Chinese doctor who was actually practising acupuncture, who had an acupuncture clinic. And I heard that he was very good. So I thought that I would give it a go. And it was after the third treatment that he gave me, that suddenly I realised that I would be able to breathe properly through my nose. He carried on for three more treatments, and I can truthfully say that my hay fever cleared up and I was virtually clear of it for about six to seven years. (Electro-acupuncturist)

Here, like the previous narratives, biomedicine is drawn upon but found wanting and there are discursive constructions that suggest a return to a pre-biomedical knowledge. The respondent states that his contact with 'an old Chinese doctor' was 'more or less out of desperation'. This clause suggests that biomedicine had failed to solve his problem, but the 'more or less' suggests that desperation was not the only reason. We can reasonably speculate that another aspect of turning to the doctor was the fact that 'I heard that he was very good' and this itself suggests that the respondent had networks linking him to this particular Chinese doctor. The respondent goes on:

Well, as things would have it, I got an appointment to work with the Hong Kong Government, and when I was there I looked around for some sort of college or some sort of institution to teach me acupuncture because I realised that there might be something in this. ... I eventually met up with a medical doctor from Shanghai ... and he taught it in a way which I could understand. He knew enough physiology and biochemistry for me to sort of latch on to, to see what was going on. ... So he had the scientific background which I felt was very necessary for me, because all the other schools of acupuncture sort of ignored that, and you are left a little bit high-and-dry, and you either believed it or not believe it and so on. (Electro-acupuncturist)

Here again we see similarities in the previous narratives. The respondent embarks upon a search and finds an approach that meets his needs. The approach he finds is one that allows him to retain his 'scientific' approach but like the others he has extended beyond the science that he was taught at medical school. Medicine is not abandoned, but the practitioners identify limitations to medicine and extend their practice beyond what the medical schools taught.

The following is from another doctor, of European ethnicity, who used a form of acupuncture:

I became interested in acupuncture in the mid-1970s, as many doctors did. There had been a sort of general movement in certain areas towards alternative medicine, not only in patients but also in practitioners. And I was with a group of young Australian doctors in the mid-1970s that became interested in acupuncture, and I have followed my interest from there. So really I started off as a medical acupuncturist doing courses that were offered under the umbrella of medical acupuncture and I have progressed, or evolved or whatever from there. ... Also I was struck as a GP of a number of years standing, before I got interested in acupuncture, the large number of cases that I, or anybody else, couldn't seem to do much about. So there was a certain amount of frustration in following the conventional approach. Frustration that not only me but other people felt. (Medical acupuncturist)

The narrative here varies to some extent from the ones we have thus far covered. In this instance the respondent positions his interest in relation to what was happening around him and what others were doing: 'a sort of general movement in certain areas towards alternative medicine'. This suggests a collective response to alternative medicine rather than simply an individual interest. This collective response has some characteristics of a social movement, where social change is not driven by the state or conventional party politics, but a popular response to social conditions. Social change is opposed to dominant norms and fosters goals of autonomy (Staggenborg 2008). Similarly, there is articulated in this narrative a collective 'frustration' at the limitations of biomedicine – 'the large number of cases that I, or anybody else, couldn't seem to do much about'. The crisis narrative articulated by previous respondents is downplayed to a narrative of frustration, but this serves a similar purpose in highlighting the limits of biomedicine and justifying the search for something beyond that provided through medical education.

The following is from a practitioner who used psychological and social approaches in practice:

I will go back to my medical school training which was back in the 1970s at Auckland. So there was an enlightened core of people there who felt that behavioural sciences should be taught to stage 3 and brought in sociologists, [and] a sort of visionary physician who talked about the value of listening to people and exploring what was going on in their lives. So we had that flavour come through the training programme but at the end of the day the biomedical model really, really was thick. And while social and psychological aspects of people's welfare was alluded to, the guts of it was that your competencies were assessed on your ability to work in a biomedical model. (Biospsychosocial practitioner)

In this narrative we have a similar structure to many of the above narratives but in a foreshortened time period. Instead of drawing on experiences in a pre-medical training life, the respondent refers to the broad vision gained in the early part of her medical training before the biomedical model overwhelmed this broad vision. The respondent goes on:

> Now I like science and I do science well and I did science well at school so
> I found med school really fascinating, but I felt increasingly uncomfortable
> when I went into my clinical years about huge chunks of people's experiences
> that just weren't being heard, and I found my clinical years from that point of
> view quite stressful. Because I could see that the consultants and the registrars
> and the whole assessment programme and the whole competency training
> programme was just not acknowledging huge chunks of people's lives. And
> in order to succeed and do well, really you had to ignore that side of yourself
> because you couldn't survive, emotionally you couldn't survive. ... I found
> my house surgeon years stressful ... you would have a patient on a ward round
> who was obviously visibly distressed and on the point of tears, and there had
> been a crisis in the family or they weren't coping about being in hospital, and
> those sorts of things never got brought up in ward rounds. (Biospsychosocial
> practitioner)

The narrative themes of the 'limits of biomedicine' and personal 'crisis' when
dealing with other people's distress is apparent. In this narrative biomedicine is
limited as, although the training is very rigorous, it does not allow practitioners to
respond to patients' concerns and experiences. More than that, if practitioners did
respond to patients' concerns and experiences they would not be able to survive
the medical training. She goes on:

> So I felt fairly disillusioned when I finished my house-surgeon years and I
> couldn't see myself working in a hospital. So I went and did the diploma of
> community medicine. ... Which was a fascinating course, and validated a lot of
> the concerns I had in my clinical school days. ... But I did miss seeing people.
> I think I realized that I actually liked working with people and seeing patients,
> so I went back to medicine and I felt a lot more confident about my perspective,
> and that is the sort of medicine I practise. I think I did practice whole-person
> medicine and patient-centred medicine but I felt very defensive about it. I
> felt very embarrassed that I included those things in my referral letters to the
> hospital. I got a lot of validation from my patients and I got some from a number
> of colleagues, but my relationship with the professional body, like hospital-
> based medicine, like 'real' medicine where specialists practise and they have the
> answers. I felt very defensive and I never felt good enough. (Biospsychosocial
> practitioner)

The narrative is of searching for a solution to the crisis and a return to views and
ideas held at an early stage – but now with a sense of security in those ideas. She
contrasts her 'whole-person medicine' with 'real' medicine of high technology
hospital-based interventions.

There are a number of clear similarities in these narratives. In no case is there
a rejection of the importance of science in medicine. In all cases there is some
point of frustration or crisis that prompts a search beyond biomedicine. For many,

what is found relates to earlier experiences or senses of identity. Becoming a better healing professional unites biomedicine with other understandings of what it takes to heal.

Discussion

The development of EBM may offer a perception that medicine is based on certainty and rigorous science, but for many medical practitioners facing everyday common problems in primary care this is not the case. Many GPs live with uncertainty in terms of diagnosis and treatment because much of what they encounter is not so easily categorised and dealt with as experimental study designs would suggest. For GPs clinical practice is complex and includes taking into account the context of patients' lives and the consequences of certain forms of diagnosis (Dew et al. 2005b). The narratives outlined in this chapter suggest that many medical practitioners turn to CAM as an EBM-dominated medical practice cannot adequately deal with this complexity. Practitioners provide a crisis narrative to explain their search for other ways of healing. A crisis narrative can be interpreted as where a moment of rupture is articulated along with a moment of transformation (Hay 1996). This transformation is frequently articulated as going from a well-educated, scientifically grounded medical practitioner to a practitioner who has decisively chosen to go beyond the limits of that education. As such they also draw on a different kind of evidential base from the narrowly defined concepts used in EBM. Evidence may be based in theory, observation and different technologies.

This crisis narrative resonates with other narratives identified in patients. In a seminal paper Bury argues that the concept of biographical disruption characterises the onset and development of chronic illness in patients. In the experience of chronic illness the disruption involves a fundamental rethinking of explanatory systems such as one's concept of oneself. It also involves a mobilisation of resources to respond to the disruption of chronic illness (Bury 1982). Other research has noted how patients facing a medical crisis, such as a diagnosis of cancer, may seek out alternatives as a way of trying to gain some control over their situation (Broom 2009a). The crisis narrative of these medical practitioners involves similar disruptions to their sense of self – as practitioners of the medical science they were taught at medical schools – and a seeking out of resources to respond to this disruption. The crisis narrative provides a warrant for these medical practitioners to extend their practices beyond the confines of standardised practices embedded within contemporary evidence-based intervention frameworks.

It could be argued that practitioners are trained in EBM so that they no longer believe in what they see before their eyes, but increasingly believe what is produced in a limited range of high impact journals and meta-analyses of interventions where a limited range of methodological approaches are accorded authority. For some who continue to believe in what they see and what they experience, CAM can offer a way out of a crisis or dilemma.

The opportunities to practice outside the narrow domain of EBM may be limited over time as centralised authorities impose standards of practice over clinicians. However, countervailing forces may also be envisaged. EBM itself may be subjected to evidential assessments and found wanting. Its narrow evidential base may lead to an expansion of the kind of methodological approaches that are given credibility in assessing healing interventions. The limitations of EBM based practice may evoke more crises stimulating practitioners to search out other forms of healing. Caution must be exercised in making generalised statements on the impact of standardisation in clinical practice and the effect on CAM. As always, there needs to be ongoing empirical study to determine what kind of impact EBM has on CAM practices.

Acknowledgments

I would like to thank Kathy Glasgow and John Gardner for their input, the medical practitioners for sharing their narratives and the editors for their helpful comments.

References

Anspach, R. 1987. Prognostic conflict in life-and-death decisions: The organization as an ecology of knowledge. *Journal of Health and Social Behaviour*, 28(3), 215–31.

Armstrong, D. 1982. The doctor–patient relationship: 1930–1980, in *The Problem of Medical Knowledge: Examining the Social Construction of Medicine*, edited by P. Wright and A. Treacher. Edinburgh: Edinburgh University Press, 109–21.

Atkinson, P. 1997. *The Clinical Experience: The Construction and Reconstruction of Clinical Reality*. Aldershot: Ashgate.

Berg, M. 1997. *Rationalizing Medical Work: Decision-support Techniques and Medical Practices*. Cambridge: MIT Press.

Bosk, C. 1986. Professional responsibility and medical error, in *Applications of Social Science to Clinical Medicine and Health Policy*, edited by L. Aiken and D. Mechanic. New Brunswick: Rutgers University Press, 460–77.

Broom, A. 2009a. 'I'd forgotten about me in all this': Discourses of self-healing, positivity and vulnerability in cancer patients' experiences of complementary and alternative medicine. *Journal of Sociology*, 45(1), 71–87.

Broom, A. 2009b. Intuition, subjectivity, and le bricoleur: Cancer patients' accounts of negotiating a plurality of therapeutic options. *Qualitative Health Research*, 19(8), 1050–59.

Bury, M. 1982. Chronic illness as biographical disruption. *Sociology of Health and Illness*, 4(2), 167–82.

Checkland, K., Harrison, S., McDonald, R., Grant, S., Campbell, S. and Guthrie, B. 2008. Biomedicine, holism and general medical practice: Responses to the 2004 General Practitioner contract. *Sociology of Health and Illness*, 30(5), 788–803.

Cochrane, A. 1972. *Effectiveness and Efficacy: Random Reflections*. London: Nuffield Provincial Hospitals Trust.

Collins, S., Britten, N., Ruusovuori, J. and Thompson, A. 1997. *Patient Participation in Health Care Consultations: Qualitative Perspectives*. Berkshire: Open University Press/McGraw Hill Education.

Dew, K. 2001. Modes of practice and models of science in medicine. *Health: An Interdisciplinary Journal for the Study of Health, Illness and Medicine*, 5(1), 93–111.

Dew, K. 2003. *Borderland Practices: Regulating Alternative Therapies in New Zealand*. Dunedin: University of Otago Press.

Dew, K. 2012 [in press]. *The Cult and Science of Health: A Sociology of Public Health*. New York: Berghahn.

Dew, K., Cumming, J., McLeod, D., Morgan, S., McKinlay, E., Dowell, A. and Love, T. 2005a. Explicit rationing of elective services: Implementing the New Zealand reforms. *Health Policy*, 74(1), 1–12.

Dew, K., Dowell, A., McLeod, D., Collings, S. and Bushnell, J. 2005b. 'This glorious twilight zone of uncertainty': Mental health consultations in general practice in New Zealand. *Social Science and Medicine*, 61(6), 1189–200.

Dew, K., Plumridge, E., Stubbe, M., Dowell, A., MacDonald, L. and Major, G. 2008. 'You just got to eat healthy': The topic of CAM in the General Practice consultation. *Health Sociology Review*, 17(4), 396–409.

Dew, K., Stubbe, M., MacDonald, L., Dowell, A. and Plumridge, E. 2010. The (non) use of prioritisation protocols by surgeons. *Sociology of Health and Illness*, 32(4), 545–62.

Dickinson, D., Wilkie, P. and Harris, M. 1999. Taking medicines: Concordance is not compliance. *British Medical Journal*, 319(7212), 787.

Eddy, D.M. 1984. Variations in physician practice: The role of uncertainty. *Health Affairs*, 3(2), 74–89.

Foucault, M. 2003. *The Birth of the Clinic: An Archaeology of Medical Perception*. London and New York: Routledge.

Glasgow, R., Vogt, T. and Boles, S. 1999. Evaluating the public health impact of health promotion interventions: The RE-AIM framework. *American Journal of Public Health*, 89(9), 1322–7.

Goodwin, D. and Mort, M. 2010. Accounting for incoherent bodies, in *Technology and Medical Practice: Blood, Guts and Machines*, edited by E. Johnson and B. Berner. Farnham: Ashgate, 51–73.

Green, J. 2000. Epistemology, evidence and experience: Evidence based health care in the work of accident alliances. *Sociology of Health and Illness*, 22(4), 453–76.

Hay, C. 1996. Narrating crisis: The discursive construction of the 'winter of discontent'. *Sociology*, 30(2), 253–77.

Henry, M. 2006. Uncertainty, responsibility, and the evolution of the physician/patient relationship. *Journal of Medical Ethics*, 32(6), 321–23.

Hess, D. 1997. *Can Bacteria Cause Cancer?* New York: New York University Press.

Klein, R., Day, P. and Redmayne, S. 1996. *Managing Scarcity: Priority Setting and Rationing in the National Health Service*. Buckingham: Open University Press.

Lipman, T. 2000. Power and influence in clinicial effectiveness and evidence-based medicine. *Family Practice*, 17(6), 557–63.

Lohr, K., Eleazer, K. and Mauskopf, J. 1998. Health policy issues and applications for evidence-based medicine and clinical practice guidelines. *Health Policy*, 46(1), 1–19.

Mead, N. and Bower, P. 2000. Patient-centredness: A conceptual framework and review of the empirical literature. *Social Science and Medicine*, 51(7), 1087–110.

Medical Council of New Zealand. 2005. *Statement on Complementary and Alternative Medicine*. [Online]. Available at: http://www.mcnz.org.nz/portals/0/guidance/comp_alternative.pdf [accessed: 19 September 2007].

Nutton, V. 2006. The rise of medicine, in *The Cambridge History of Medicine*, edited by R. Porter. Cambridge: Cambridge University Press, 46–70.

Petryna, A. 2007. Clinical trials offshored: On private sector science and public health. *BioSocieties*, 2, 21–40.

Polich, G., Dole, C. and Kaptchuk, T. 2010. The need to act a little more 'scientific': Biomedical researchers investigating complementary and alternative medicine. *Sociology of Health and Illness*, 32(1), 106–22.

Porter, R. 2006. Hospitals and surgery, in *The Cambridge History of Medicine*, edited by R. Porter. Cambridge: Cambridge University Press, 176–210.

Porter, T. 1995. *Trust in Numbers: The Pursuit of Objectivity in Science and Public Life*. Princeton: Princeton University Press.

Rhodes, P., Langdon, M., Rowley, E., Wright, J. and Small, N. 2006. What does the use of a computerized checklist mean for patient-centred care? The example of a routine diabetes review. *Qualitative Health Research*, 16(3), 353–76.

Rosenthal, M. 1995. *The Incompetent Doctor: Behind Closed Doors*. Buckingham: Open University Press.

Scott, J. 1998. *Seeing Like a State: How Certain Schemes to Improve the Human Condition Have Failed*. New Haven and London: Yale University Press.

Smith, R. 1991. Where is the wisdom. *British Medical Journal*, 393(6806), 798–9.

Staggenborg, S. 2008. *Social Movements*. Oxford: Oxford University Press.

Timmermans, S. and Berg, M. 2003. *The Gold Standard: The Challenge of Evidence-based Medicine and Standardization in Health Care*. Philadelphia: Temple University Press.

Wallis, K. 2009. Uncertainty, fear, and whistling happy tunes. *Journal of Primary Health Care*, 1(1), 71–3.

Weber, M. 1948. *From Max Weber*. London: Routledge and Kegan Paul.

Willis, E. and White, K. 2004. Evidence-based medicine and CAM, in *The Mainstreaming of Complementary and Alternative Medicine*, edited by P. Tovey, G. Easthope and J. Adams. London and New York: Routledge, 49–63.

Chapter 8

Patient Understandings of Evidence and Therapeutic Effectiveness

Alex Broom and Philip Tovey

Introduction

Increasingly the second wave of EBHC has emphasised patient perspectives, evidence-based patient choice and evidence-based patient care. At least at the level of policy and representation, there has been a movement away from an emphasis on distanced cohort data with increased attention given to the applicability of data for individual patients and clinical contexts. Despite this, as Holmes and O'Byrne emphasise in Chapter 3, EBM and EBP have remained reliant on epidemiological data and reductive approaches to care regardless of linguistic and rhetorical shifts. It is for this reason that we place this chapter in Part III ('Evidence on the Margins') rather than in Part II ('Evidence in the Clinic'). Whilst this is perhaps slightly provocative – there is some penetration of patient views on evidence into clinical environments – patient understandings of what constitutes effectiveness have been consistently marginalised. As shown in the data presented below, while patient perspectives are continuing to shape clinical work and clinical practices, they often vary significantly from those of biomedical clinicians and EBM/EBP advocates. A refocusing on what patients themselves understand as evidence becomes an inevitable conclusion.

In this chapter we ask British patients themselves 'what is evidence?' and in a particularly controversial context: the use of complementary and alternative medicine (CAM) in the context of cancer. There is perhaps no more divisive a public and academic debate than that of the use of CAM in the treatment of cancer and such debates tend to feature those operating at the extremes of the 'evidence debate' (that is, those espousing meta-analysis of clinical trials versus those who treat on the basis of individual need). This very public debate has largely focused on the 'lack of proof' discourse espoused by CAM sceptics rather than the 'lack of a need for proof' discourse of CAM advocates. While there are stakeholders pursuing a more nuanced position, there has been little movement in the area of CAM and cancer in terms of health policy or health delivery in the UK. Most CAM use for cancer is private, making it a fascinating case study of patient decision making taking place outside conventional medicine facilities and involving considerations around what works and what constitutes evidence of effectiveness.

Below we interrogate how 80 cancer patients view, make sense of, and process, issues related to evidence. That is, how they decide what constitutes an effective treatment, how they negotiate what constitutes evidence with their clinicians, and how they make sense of disjunctions between what they believe and what others say is true. The aim of this chapter is to unpack a group of British cancer patients' perspectives on the nature of evidence and the degree to which different understandings of evidence inform decision making about CAM and biomedicine. In addressing this aim, the chapter explores the complexities surrounding the move to evidence-based models of care. We note at this point that the current trajectory in British cancer care is toward the creation of a biomedical-type evidence base to inform both decisions on funding and patient decision making. This, many argue, will ensure that patients are able to avoid 'ineffective' treatments. We argue here that while cancer patients may indeed appreciate the nature of scientific evidence *per se*, and its usefulness in certain scenarios, many also perceive scientific evidence to be highly inadequate for measuring effectiveness and thus predicting how their body will respond to treatment. As such, here we provide a conceptual model of patient perspectives on evidence that we consider must inform the trajectory of EBHC in the twenty-first century.

Patient Support for Complementary Medicine and the Challenges it Presents for EBM

The rise of CAM has been a significant development within healthcare over the last three decades with CAM therapies increasingly popular among a wide range of patient groups (Cassileth and Vickers 2005). The widespread popularity of CAM in the UK has raised the question of the potential integration of CAM into UK cancer services. However, despite national cancer policy increasingly advocating 'integrative' and 'patient-centred' practice (Department of Health 2000, 2004), a virtual stalemate in debate about evidence and efficacy has prevented any real progress being made. Many biomedical stakeholders argue for the development of a biomedical-type evidence base prior to the consideration of including CAM therapies into the National Health Service (NHS) (Ernst 2001). However, an increasingly popular perspective amongst CAM practitioners, patient groups and some social scientists alike, is that, professional gate-keeping, paradigmatic incommensurability and restrictive understandings of evidence are the real barriers to state funding of CAM (Borgerson 2005, Broom and Tovey 2007). Moreover, patients themselves are increasingly choosing treatments regardless of their clinical efficacy (Lewith, Broomfield and Prescott 2002). This behaviour suggests that the pursuit of evidence-based medicine may not resonate with many patients' experiences.

What is CAM?

There is considerable debate over what CAM is and what characterises CAM practices; issues well covered in existing sociological literature (Broom 2002). To contextualise the following discussion it is important to emphasise that CAM is a constructed and dynamic entity that is historically and culturally variable. It refers to a diverse and often paradigmatically disparate range of therapeutic practices. Broadly, the category 'CAM' is used to refer to a wide range of therapeutic practices including: aromatherapy, naturopathy, herbalism, homeopathy, reiki, acupuncture and spiritual healing. Whilst acknowledging the complexities outlined above, there are certain parallels we can draw between CAMs. What largely characterises CAMs is, first, a lack of integration into western health care systems and, second, their tendency to espouse models of care that incorporate physical and metaphysical elements in treatment processes. There is also some merit, as shall be illustrated later, in distinguishing between 'whole systems' approaches like naturopathy or homeopathy and the less ideologically-driven healing approaches such as reiki, aromatherapy massage or healing touch.

CAM and Evidence

As discussed in Chapter 7, critiques of biomedicine have often centred on the highly positivist ontological framework imposed by the biomedical model and the epistemological biases inherent in knowledge produced through RCTs (Borgerson 2005). The RCT, some argue, provides a highly restrictive view of the therapeutic process and is gauged towards measuring reductionistic notions of effectiveness. Through the imposition of a disease-centred (rather than patient-centred) framework, CAMs have been viewed by many as unproven, whereas, it is often argued by advocates, the therapeutic processes involved in CAM practices cannot be adequately captured in a positivist framework (Borgerson 2005). This has led some to focus on more patient-centred and subjective gauges of validity including notions of wellbeing, healing and achieving balance.

Efforts to prompt biomedical organisations and clinicians to critically engage in debates about evidence production and address complex ideological and paradigmatic issues have been largely unsuccessful. A major schism persists between critics and proponents of CAM – a schism that largely settles on the issue of evidence.

CAM and Cancer

Despite difficulties in defining CAM, we can provide some indication of the extent of usage. Bringing together 26 surveys from 13 countries, Ernst and Cassileth

(1998) found that on average 31.4 per cent of cancer patients use CAM therapies. UK surveys show similar figures with over 30 per cent of people with cancer reporting use (Lewith, Broomfield and Prescott 2002). Results vary across cancer types. Morris et al. (2000) found that breast cancer patients were most likely to be users, suggesting variability between patients with different cancer types and/ or according to gender. Although little research has been done to tease out such issues, it seems possible that type of cancer, demographics, available treatments, symptoms and rate of progression may each have an influence on patients' preferences for CAM.

Postmodernisation, Reflexivity and Technologies of the Self

Over the last two decades sociologists have engaged in debates about the implications of increased pluralism in healthcare, and indeed, the character of different forms of practice, evidence and knowledge production. Sociological research on CAM has drawn on a range of theoretical traditions to conceptualise developments, with numerous attempts made at linking CAM use to: a societal shift to postmodernity; processes of reflexive modernisation; and, the emergence of new forms of selfhood. As we shall illustrate, these conceptual arguments have often been speculatively linked to grand theory with little grounding in empirical data.

The postmodernisation thesis has been popular amongst some CAM sociologists as an explanation for the increased presence of CAM. Its proponents view CAM use as reflecting wider patterns related to the postmodernisation of social life (Bakx 1991, Eastwood 2000, Rayner and Easthope 2001, Siahpush 1998). In this context postmodernisation is broadly seen to denote an increased fragmentation of experience, consumerism, individualisation and aestheticisation of social life. In the context of healthcare, metanarratives (such as the biomedical model) are subsumed by subjective individualised knowledges that inform social practices and identity work. CAM use, within this model, is viewed as a rejection of metanarratives related to disease and the selection, and production, of individualised understandings of disease and treatment regimes. Implicit in such arguments is the increased prioritisation of lay knowledges of disease, and importantly, the rejection of the superiority of scientific knowledge and expertise. While this theory has been widely drawn on, its applicability has been seriously questioned in recent scholarship and it is a theoretical position that has rarely been subject to empirical investigation (Tovey, Atkin and Milewa 2001).

Social theorisations of late modernity have also been drawn on in attempts to conceptualise patients' preferences for CAM (Low 2004, Tovey, Atkin and Milewa 2001). Moving beyond the rather over simplistic 'fragmentation of experience' and 'individualisation' themes implicit in the postmodernisation thesis, authors like Beck (1992) and Giddens (1991) have focused on increased reflexivity in modern societies and the tendency of consumers to be more critical of expert knowledges. The result, it has been argued, is that people have become more sceptical of the judgements or advice of (scientific) experts (Lupton and Tulloch 2002), actively assessing the merits of particular claims. This in turn, it has been postulated, has opened up the potential for the proliferation of CAM – a backlash against the perceived failings of science and biomedical technologies (Kaptchuk and Eisenberg 1998).

There have also been recent attempts to theorise the potential implications, at an individual level, of new therapeutic models of care for changing notions of selfhood (Doel and Segrott 2003, Sointu 2006). This work has examined the degree to which CAM use represents a significant shift in conceptions of disease and selfhood. In particular, the notion of wellbeing has emerged recently as a potentially useful concept for characterising what CAM offers to the individual. Departing from biomedical notions of being cured, healthy or disease-free, wellbeing encapsulates notions of authenticity, recognition and self-determination; restructuring health as a subjective and individualised process (Bishop and Yardley 2004, Sointu 2006). CAM use is thus conceptualised as a project that reproduces the self – an individual search for recognition as being an authentic self that is both discovered by the individual and shaped by the nature of individual therapeutic practices.

Social theorisations of wellbeing have emphasised the limitations of biomedical conceptions of disease and health, and are thus, in part, a conceptual extension of the depersonalisation (McClean 2005) and deindividualisation (Anspach 1988) theses. These two latter arguments refer broadly to processes by which many biomedical clinicians abstract from the individual through speech (such as referring to 'the patient'), technologies (such as viewing the person as a biomedicalised image), statistical probabilities (such as the group rather than individual), units of analysis (e.g. genes/cellular) and so on, rather than acknowledging the individual subject. This is seen to alienate the patient from treatment processes – perhaps even resulting in the need for alternative therapeutic options.

As illustrated above, sociological theory as applied to CAM has tended to engage in the reification of broader sociocultural shifts in relation to individual choice, conceptions of disease and lay–expert relations. Rather than reflecting broad paradigmatic change, we argue that that the increasing presence of CAM in cancer care should be characterised as a dialectical tension between therapeutic processes engendering individuation (for example through an emphasis on agency, self-responsibility, wellbeing and individual healing) and depersonalisation (for example through an emphasis on cure rates, probabilities and abstraction). That is, tensions between different forms of knowledge (tacit, intuitive, formalised, encoded) and evidence of effectiveness (trial based, experiential, learnt). Moreover, we argue here that the ways in which patients attempt to manage this individuation/depersonalisation dialectic is deeply embedded in the nature of their disease (that is, disease stage and prognosis) and age.

Fieldwork

This study involved NHS teaching hospitals and one partially NHS-funded hospice in the north of England. Two cancer specialists and a CAM coordinator at the hospice who had formed part of the project team assisted with recruitment. This project was a 30-month qualitative study utilising in-depth interviews. The final sample included 80 cancer patients with a good distribution of ages from 20 to 87 and representation from all major cancer types and stages of disease. A third of the participants were male whereas two thirds were female. The number of excerpts presented in the results broadly reflects this differential. Given the high proportion of female CAM users reported in previous studies we had expected to recruit more female participants. Interestingly, despite a gender split in uptake of CAM, number of women in the sample and the types of therapies used, there was no evidence that gender significantly impacted on the dialectic discussed in the results.

Of the sample, 68 were white British. The remaining 12 were Irish (4), Indian (2), Italian (2), German (2) and Eastern European (2). The majority were CAM users although 12 non-CAM users were interviewed in order to gain some insight into perceptions of CAM and evidence from a range of perspectives. We deliberately sampled in such a way as to include high numbers of CAM users in order to gain insight into experiences of CAM and biomedicine in relation to evidence. Thus, this is a study of predominantly CAM users who are cancer patients rather than a representative sample of all cancer patients; this recognition informed our interpretation of the results.

All the respondents were interviewed in either their own homes, their oncology ward, at the hospice or at the authors' university, for between one to two hours. With the permission of the participant, the interviews were audio-recorded and subsequently fully transcribed. The interviews were relatively unstructured, exploring: patients' understandings of, and beliefs about, evidence; how effectiveness is talked about in relation to CAM and the importance of different forms of knowledge, actors and institutional processes play in these accounts; and, the influence of different forms of evidence in patients' perceptions, and usage, of CAM. The aim was to achieve a detailed understanding of the varying positions adhered to and to locate these within an appreciation of broader underlying beliefs and agendas. The approach we used was developmental in that knowledge generated in the early interviews was challenged, compared with, and built upon by later ones.

Lay Perspectives on Scientific Evidence

A central issue for this study was to achieve an understanding of the ways these cancer patients' view scientific evidence and the conceptual basis of their assessments of the legitimacy of scientific knowledge in decision-making.

Participants' responses were quite varied. However, what was clear was that a significant number of these patients viewed evidence and scientific knowledge as highly problematic concepts. Moreover, their views regarding the nature of evidence production were often closely linked with their use of non-biomedical treatments:

P: It is very difficult to get any information on [ovarian cancer] apart from statistics and how many folk die with [ovarian cancer] and that wasn't what I wanted, that wasn't what I needed. ... I mean, they [doctors] are not God, they don't know how long somebody has got to live, I don't care who they are. ... Some people get given a prognosis and they will live. The statistics take away something if you listen to them. They take away hope ... your own ability to heal yourself. (Female, 58 years, ovarian, metastatic)

Another respondent:
I: How important is scientific evidence for you?

P: Not particularly. I don't think so, because, as medicine itself is an interaction between the individual and what you are giving them. ... So, you could take 100 people and it might not work for 70 of them, but if they are not working with it, that is why it is not working ... also, you personally haven't got a 70 per cent chance of cure anyway. It's that 70 per cent of people will be cured, that's different isn't it? (Female, 51 years, bowel, metastatic disease)

Another respondent:
P: Science can only take you so far. I'm a religious person so I'm quite spiritual so there's all that side of things and there's evidence from your own experience which you may not be able to write down in a formula. So, I mean ... I don't care; it's not the be all and end all what science says, although I respect it. (Female, 70 years, ovarian, metastatic disease)

As illustrated above, a significant proportion of these patients, regardless of whether they had opted to use CAMs or not, had ambivalent (if not negative) feelings towards statistics and probabilities on cure. Given the fact that most were still undergoing treatment, whether for potentially curable or metastatic disease, they were faced with the difficult task of trying to decide who to trust. Moreover, they each attempted to critically assess the paradigmatic basis of the knowledge that was being given to them, often coming up with complex critiques of different forms of knowledge. Biomedicine was not, in large part, considered flawed as a discipline, nor were statistics viewed as having no use. In fact, most of these patients acknowledged that statistics were accurate in terms of how the average number of people will react to a particular treatment. However, a significant proportion felt that this told them little about how they personally would react to treatment. Lifestyle, emotion and spirituality were often described as factors that may heavily influence whether you were, for example, in the 70 per cent who were cured or the 30 per cent who were not.

Illustrated in the second excerpt shown above, a common view was that it was not that one had a certain percentage chance of survival, but rather, it was that a certain percentage of people would survive. Initially this seems like splitting hairs, but in fact, it vividly illustrates what many participants felt biomedical statistics could not give them – concrete knowledge about how they, a unique individual, would react to treatment. Statistics were viewed as a crude conglomerate of disparate bodies and unique lives. Thus, although biomedical evidence was viewed as being able to accurately show effectiveness over the wider patient population, it was not viewed as being able to show the effectiveness of a treatment for a specific individual.

As is shown later, this logic was also crucial in terms of decisions to utilise CAM. For some, their experience of biomedical decision-making processes led them to develop a critical view of medical statistics and to seek out and use CAMs. For others, critiques of biomedical knowledge had been learnt from their CAM practitioner/s and were deployed to justify their decision making in relation to biomedicine (or their rejection of their prognosis). In such cases, CAM therapists had employed ideological critiques of biomedical statistics to justify the lack of evidence that existed to back up their own treatments and the individual patient would utilise this framework to make sense of the legitimacy of the CAM therapy and the restrictive nature of their prognosis (this is expanded on below).

It is important to emphasise that patients' views of evidence were embedded in, but not dictated by, the nature of their disease, stage and prognosis. It was acknowledged by several of the patients that the better the statistical probability was for cure, regardless of the flaws inherent in the application of statistics to the individual, the less likely it was to be a bad result for the individual. Thus, their critiques of biomedical statistics, perhaps unsurprisingly, were very much linked to feelings of ambiguity about the result:

> P: One is hardly going to argue about cure rates when faced with a 90 per cent chance of cure. You'd say, 'Thank God for that'. You really only start to question statistics when they aren't going your way. Or, I suppose, when it [the treatment outcome] could go either way. Also, what they say [CAM therapists] is also going to be more appealing I suppose.

> *Later in the interview:*
> P: I must say, I am more critical [of science] now than earlier [before treatment]. Of course I thought the result would be a lot better than it was. (Female, 45 years, breast, metastatic)

In certain situations, impressive success rates require little consideration of other factors that may play a role in healing, or indeed, enlisting alternative models of healing. This was illustrated in the accounts of some of the patients with localised tumours or curable metastatic disease who were told they had an excellent chance of cure. Thus, patients' perceptions of, and tendency to critically assess, biomedical evidence were very much embedded in the 'odds' they were given and how acceptable they felt these were. The more ambiguous or negative the 'odds' became, the more statistics were viewed as unable to predict. Moreover, the degree to which the prognosis was acceptable seemed to be mediated by age.

Whereas the younger patients tended to have real difficulty accepting their prognosis; older patients often experienced fewer problems accepting a prognosis of around, say, a five-year survival. As one 73 year-old male with prostate cancer said: 'I've had a pretty good run so far so I'm not bothered really'. In such cases, patients were less likely to question prognostic data, use whole system CAMs or develop critiques of biomedical knowledge. This, it would seem, may also be connected to (potentially hegemonic) discourses of ageing and perceptions of coming to a 'natural end' rather than the need to 'fight' and 'get well':

> P: I was very interested in my son's cancer. ... I really wanted to know all about that but I never really cared about [my cancer] and finding out information. I thought, I'm older, this is my lot. I mean he's younger; it was a big tragedy you know. (Female, 70 years, ovarian, metastatic)

Thus, it may be the case that the need to challenge one's prognosis and question evidence (and in fact, potentially utilise CAMs) is embedded in wider cultural constructions of the appropriateness of sickness or indeed cure for certain age groups and types of individuals. In saying this, as is illustrated later in our discussion, the younger cancer patients interviewed have grown up in the context of a relative waning in deference to biomedical expertise. Thus, these intersecting but also distinct factors (that is age and medico-cultural context) potentially mediate these patients' perceptions of evidence and CAM as well as their tendency to accept or question their actual prognosis.

It also emerged from the interviews that 'what is rational' is very much situated, in that, when faced with a terminal illness, people will question established knowledge that otherwise they would not. This was not viewed as an act of desperation, but critical thinking at a pivotal point in life:

> P: These people that sit there saying, 'How do you believe in these therapies?' They are not where we are. Have any of these people got terminal cancer or a terminal disease? They aren't in that position, so they don't know, it's like anything, as much as you commiserate, you do not really fully understand what it's like ... you have got to be in that position to fully understand how it feels ... and if you were in this position, you'd get out there and try things. (Female, 58 years, ovarian, metastatic)

Another respondent:
> I: As your prognosis changed, did your need for complementary therapies?

P: I think, yes, obviously I have moved more that way now because they
     [medical specialists] are not offering me much anymore, so I am prepared
     to give it a go ... and you question whether what they say [medical
     specialists] is really true. (Female, 51 years, bowel, advanced)

These patients' critiques of science, biomedical knowledge and utilisation
of CAMs, in this context, could be construed as a response to the uncertainty
of an ambiguous diagnosis and indeed, these patients were fully aware of this
discourse of CAM use. As illustrated in the second excerpt above, some of these
patients recall making a deliberate decision to investigate non-biomedical options
and question biomedical statistics as their prognosis worsened; an illustration of
how perceptions evolve over the disease process. However, although fear and
uncertainty undoubtedly contribute to perceptions of scientific evidence and
alternative models of care, decision-making processes are much more complex
and cannot be reduced to a need for hope in the face of death. Rather, critiques
of depersonalisation and abstraction and the value placed in the attributes of
alternative forms (and models of) cancer care, need to be placed in a wider context
of the need for subjectivity, agency and self-determination in disease and treatment
processes.

Agency, Subjectivity and Self-Determination

Participants' critiques of biomedical evidence tended to espouse a highly
individualised view of disease and treatment response. These reflections were
sometimes drawn from their interactions with CAM practitioners. For other
patients, critiques of this kind of evidence were the product of working through
their emotions in relation to medical statistics and interactions with biomedical
clinicians. Regardless of the origin of the critique, such feelings were characterised
by a strong desire to retain their own subjectivity and self-determination. Statistics,
in many cases, were seen to demoralise and take away 'hope'.

Scientific evidence and biomedical treatment processes were seen to limit
human agency, produce anxiety, and in extreme cases even induce death as patients
choose to 'give up on life'. The imposition of the collective (or depersonalisation)
on the individual was viewed, in such cases, as an unethical and ultimately
counter-productive practice employed by many biomedical clinicians. In response
to the threat of statistics on cure rates, a number of the patients (although a
distinct minority) refused to be told their prognosis. Although, in part, this was
probably also about not wanting to hear potentially 'bad news', probability was
seen to impose abstracted and oversimplified patterns on a subjective and unique
individual (McClean 2005).

For significant numbers of the patients with metastatic disease, their CAM
practitioners often played a pivotal role in ensuring they had 'hope' and in
countering their feelings of despondency resulting from their prognosis. Patients

would develop a critique of biomedical evidence from conversations with their individual practitioner about the prognosis; a process that could be construed as CAM practitioners leading patients away from legitimate biomedical knowledge. However, if we look closer we see that patients place high value on certain facets of alternative approaches to treatment – a value that cannot be reduced to a 'desperate' need for hope when faced by a negative prognosis:

I: For you, in deciding whether to use a treatment or not, how important is the existence of scientific evidence?

P: Quite important, although when I first started to see [name of CAM practitioner] and I spoke to other people about it, they always put an emphasis on what his results were like – the percentage of success rate. So often I ask [name of CAM practitioner] and he would say, 'Patients that I cure is 100% success rate, patients that I don't is a 0% success rate'. That would annoy me a bit because, well, that's not an answer, but what I realised is, how can he have these statistics, you have to look at cases, individual cases, you can't just put a figure at the end of it – a 70 per cent success rate. (Male, 25 years, LP nodular hodgkins, metastatic)

Another respondent:

I: How important is scientific evidence for you?

P: Well, if [patients] are not working with [the treatment], that is why it is not working. It's not the therapy that is not working; it's the interaction between the individual and the therapy that is not working. Medical studies are always done at arms' length, so really, your interaction with the people who are giving you the medicine is not considered, it's just irrelevant. So, I think the evidence is whether it works for you. (Female, 51 years, bowel, metastatic)

Another respondent:

P: I just think, no, sorry, you might not be able to equate it [CAM therapy]; you may not be able to put any sort of balance on it and say that it is researchable, quantifiable or whatever, but yes, I just believe it works. (Female, 40 years, adrenal, metastatic)

Again we see how these patients, and many of the others interviewed, conceptualised evidence in relation to CAM. It was not that they rejected outright the ability of statistics to tell them useful things about the successes of biomedical and CAM cancer treatments for a group; it is that science was not perceived to be able to predict what would happen to them and to their body.

As we see in the first excerpt, such critiques of statistics and scientisation were often encouraged by their CAM practitioners who also drew on highly individualised understandings of illness and the body. We see this again in the following description of a spiritual healer's approach:

> P: She reckoned the reason which I had got cancer, was because my chakras
> were not working … it was about a lack of energy balance in my body. …
> It's totally different to the way doctors work … they [CAM practitioners]
> focus on your [emphasis] life and your individual stuff and not just the
> disease and statistics. (Male, 27 years, testicular, post-curative)

As a discipline, clinical epidemiology emerged as a method of ensuring that the clinician and the patient have a high degree of certainty about the effects of an intervention – all things being equal, processes of randomisation are designed to produce accurate chances of treatment success. As suggested by a number of the patients interviewed here, this very process of randomisation and abstraction may also obscure the impact of the individual on their body and disease.

The discourse of individuality is complicated by the fact that often these patients genuinely desired statistics to defend their use of a particular CAM practitioner to family and friends. At the same time, critiques of evidence were appealing given the fact that they appreciated the highly subjective nature of the treatment process and the importance of the individual in shaping the treatment outcome. In this sense, we have a complex combination of a prognosis, a desire for cure, but also a need for a paradigm which gives hope and a sense of control over one's fate.

It is important to note that the characteristics of the CAMs being used also potentially shapes patients' perspectives on evidence and biomedical care. Some of the practices used by these patients can be characterised as whole systems approaches like herbalism, homeopathy or naturopathy. Whereas these therapeutic systems seek to treat the patient's cancer or symptomatology, other CAM practices such as healing touch or reiki may merely seek to alleviate pain or psychological distress. The latter practices also tend to involve limited discussion of ideology, whereas in the case of the whole systems approaches, discussion of the paradigmatic basis of the treatment can be both a crucial part of the client–practitioner encounter and play a central role in shaping patients' perspectives on biomedical cancer care. As one patient recalled of her spiritual healer:

> She said not to worry about why it works but to let it work. She said she just
> helps the conventional treatments do their job and that's all. She made no claims
> to cure or anything. … I don't think she liked that I had been told there was no
> hope for me but … she wasn't going to push me away from [doctors] … she
> wouldn't criticise them either. (Female, breast, metastatic)

Thus, we can see that the character of the individual CAM user and the CAMs they utilise each potential influence the propensity to critique scientific knowledge and biomedical prognoses.

Experiential Knowledge, CAM Therapies and Trust in Science

Dissatisfaction with biomedical science and statistics on cure rates often led these patients to try things out and pursue a trajectory whereby they would purely judge a treatment on the outcome rather than its philosophy or available statistical evidence. In some cases, patients had already used the particular type of CAM previously for a minor illness (for example homeopathic or herbal remedies) but most of the time patients merely tried out treatments they had heard of before but had never actually used. One patient described this process as a 'leap of faith' whereby the patient largely ignores the 'logic' behind the treatment:

> P: The things that I could see, I could see with healing, I could see physically
>   that it was working. I could see that with the trances and the physical
>   reactions that she [spiritual healer] was having in the room. So you couldn't
>   prove that scientifically but I knew it was working. And the thing is, when
>   she sort of recommended the crystals, because I knew the other things were
>   working, I sort of went along with it really. I didn't understand scientifically
>   how the crystals actually worked and ... I wasn't really interested. (Male, 27
>   years, testicular, post-curative)

What emerged was a significant group of cancer patients prioritising experiential knowledge and rejecting the need for scientific evidence in treatment decisions. Some of the CAMs used including spiritual healing and psychic surgery involved, what some would consider, quite exotic practices, but yet these patients chose to judge the therapies on their effect rather than the basis of the practice itself. For many respondents, the science behind the treatments was irrelevant and feeling 'better in myself' was the ultimate measure of whether a treatment was working or not.

The prioritising of experiential knowledge and scepticism toward science seemed closely linked to various historical events that were perceived to reflect the dangers of trusting expert opinion and scientific knowledge. Moreover, the willingness to experiment and try alternatives was shown in the interviews to be embedded in a wider sociohistorical context of waning trust in scientific expertise:

> I: To you how important is scientific evidence?

> P: Not really, it's not important whatsoever. I'm now 57 and I see that many
>   experts come out with so many wonderful ideas and then a few years later it
>   come as how it's a total load of rubbish ... like the big thing about GM
>   foods, is it good or is it no good? If somebody in a white coat was to tell me
>   something I wouldn't take it as God's gospel ... I just try it and see if it
>   works for me. (Male, 57 years, bowel, post-curative)

A number of patients felt that their ability to trust medical experts had been eroded by various medical controversies and perceived misinformation given to the public over the dangers of particular drugs and diseases. Thalidomide, genetically modified food and mad cow disease were often used as examples of the fallibility of medical advice and the need to make one's own assessments of both risk and benefit.

However, views of evidence and scientific knowledge were not linear. In fact, some patients rejected all forms of knowledge that did not draw on scientific method. As perhaps could be expected, these tended to be the non-CAM users in the study, although, we should emphasise that CAM use was not a determining factor:

> P: I would never dream of giving up conventional medicine and my drugs. And, whatever they [the doctors] say to me, I do. Whatever they [doctors] say. If they say go and sit in a hot bath for three hours, I'd go and sit in a hot bath because I believe what they say. That's normal, I mean, why would you not? (Female, 69 years, uterus, metastatic)

Another respondent:
> P: I am a bit wary … I have read about things like the Gerson diet, and, I mean, they don't work. They die these people and to do something that is so radical without the proof that it works … no! [exclamation]. I need proof. (Female, 53 years, leukaemia, metastatic)

Although a minority in the overall sample, there were a number of patients who gave full support to the superiority of scientific knowledge. For these patients it was a matter of unconditional trust in the sense that they would do absolutely anything their specialist told them to do. From this perspective, biomedicine had the best track record of success; the most rigorous research methods; and, was most ethical in their claims-making. Thus, we see a spectrum of views of evidence and the legitimacy of biomedical knowledge within this study, emphasising the importance of a policy trajectory that also acknowledges significant differentiation in patients' views of, and desire for, a biomedical type evidence-base.

Discussion

In this chapter we have presented an empirical and conceptual examination of the ways in which a group of 80 cancer patients conceptualise and utilise different forms of evidence in relation to CAM and biomedicine. Through their stories of care and illness have illustrated that what CAM achieves for individual patients is not linear and patients' perceptions, and utilisation, of different forms of evidence (scientific or otherwise) vary considerably according to the individual patient's ontological and epistemological positioning (which are in turn mediated by their disease and treatment trajectories).

Alternative models of healing are valued, primarily, for their subjectified (rather than abstracted) and individualised (rather than depersonalised) approach to cancer care; an approach that was seen to allow for, and promote, agency, self-determination and ultimately hope. CAM practitioners were seen by many of those interviewed to promote a 'project of the self'; a reclaiming of hope, subjectivity and control – elements that were largely perceived to be neglected in biomedical cancer care. Particularly in cases of uncertainty and ambiguity about success rates, statistical probabilities were perceived to create an environment of determinism that promoted fatalism. There was not a rejection of the value of biomedical statistics, but rather, a critical view which emphasised their limited scope and weakness for predicting outcomes for the individual patient.

Cancer represents a highly specific context in which the consumption of CAM has particular meanings (and serves particular roles); meanings that may be very different than those observed in other disease and health contexts. The threat of terminal illness clearly has considerable implications for patients' preparedness to extend beyond traditional notions of evidence and effectiveness; moreover, therapeutic approaches that promote indeterminacy ('my fate is unclear') and self-determination ('I can make a difference') are going to be extremely appealing for many patients who have metastatic or advanced disease.

Ultimately most of the patients interviewed here still considered that biomedical knowledge and expertise play an important role in their cancer care, regardless of the difficulties they had with evidence and statistical probabilities. Thus, at least within this context, the notions of a broader paradigm shift (postmodernity), increasing distrust in science (reflexive modernisation) or the emergence of a forms of identity work (individual wellbeing), alone, do not capture the complexity of these patients' engagement with CAM and biomedicine. Although these conceptual arguments each provide some insight into what is a complex social phenomenon, what characterises these patients' engagement with CAM in cancer care is a complex dialectical tension between the appeal of individualisation (recognition of the subjective self) and depersonalisation (appeal of control and certainty) – a tension that for most patients is not actually resolved but rather managed through the disease and treatment processes.

The management of this dialectic – or indeed the appeal of these ontological extremes – were shown in this study to be inextricably tied to these patients' own desire for (and thus the attraction of) particular ontological and epistemological positions within the management of their specific disease. Thus, we advocate a theoretical approach that acknowledges both the emerging dialectic between individuation and depersonalisation, but also the role of physiological and demographic factors (for example age) which influence how individual patients attempt to resolve such tensions.

Conclusion

UK cancer policy is largely driven by a need for a biomedical-type evidence base. That is, if it isn't proven in a trial it will not be provided to patients within the NHS. This is regardless of patient support or need. While CAM practices, not proven in the biomedical sense are being allowed in through the volunteer sector and through initiatives at specific hospitals, NHS structures and the Department of Health policies largely exlude CAM practices on the basis on evidence (or lack thereof) (Broom and Tovey, 2007). This policy and practice trajectory does not acknowledge the kinds of ontological and epistemological complexities that British cancer patients themselves engage with such as: what constitutes evidence for me, in my life; does abstract biomedical knowledge apply to the individual; and, exactly who (and what) decides what constitutes legitimate knowledge of disease and treatment processes? As illustrated in these patients' accounts, decision-making about CAM is mediated by a range of complex personal and social processes and scientific evidence may or may not play an influential role in decision-making. This is largely a reflection of the fact that many cancer patients seem acutely aware of the contingent and ultimately multifaceted nature of evidence and knowledge of the body.

We conclude, therefore, that the production of a biomedical-type evidence base for CAM, will in all likelihood have little influence on cancer patients' views of, and decisions to use, CAM. Indeed health policy more broadly must reflect the types of complex issues that patients face in decision making and treatment processes including the multifaceted nature of the notions of evidence and effectiveness.

Acknowledgements

This project was funded by a Department of Health Research and Development Grant (09/02). We thank the patients for their willingness to participate in this project at a time of significant emotional and physical challenge. Parts of this chapter were originally published in the journal *Sociology*, 41(6), 1021–39. Reprinted by Permission of SAGE.

References

Anspach, R. 1988. Notes on the sociology of medical discourse. *Journal of Health and Social Behaviour*, 29(4), 357–75.
Bakx, K. 1991 The 'eclipse' of folk medicine in western society. *Sociology of Health and Illness*, 13(1), 20–38.
Beck, U. 1992. *Risk Society*. London: Sage.

Bishop, F. and Yardley, L. 2004. Constructing agency in treatment decisions. *Health*, 8(4), 465–82.

Borgerson, K. 2005. Evidence-based alternative medicine? *Perspectives in Biology and Medicine*, 48(4), 502–15.

Broom, A. 2002. Contested territories: The construction of boundaries between 'alternative' and 'conventional' cancer treatments. *New Zealand Journal of Sociology*, 17(2), 215–34.

Broom, A. and Tovey, P. 2007. Therapeutic pluralism? Evidence, power and legitimacy in UK cancer services. *Sociology of Health and Illness*, 29(3), 551–69.

Cassileth, B. and Vickers, A. 2005. High prevalence of complementary and alternative medicine use among cancer patients. *Journal of Clinical Oncology*, 23(12), 2590–92.

Department of Health. 2000. *NHS Cancer Plan*. London: Department of Health.

Department of Health. 2004. *The NHS Cancer Plan and the New NHS*. London: Department of Health.

Doel, M. and Segrott, J. 2003. Self, health, and gender: Complementary and alternative medicine in the British mass media. *Gender, Place and Culture*, 10(2), 131–44.

Eastwood, H. 2000. Why are Australian GPs using alternative medicine? Postmodernisation, consumerism and the shift towards holistic health. *Journal of Sociology*, 36(2) 133–55.

Ernst, E. and Cassileth, S. 1998. The prevalence of complementary/alternative medicine in cancer: A systematic review. *Cancer*, 83(4), 777–82.

Ernst, E. 2001. *The Desktop Guide to CAM*. Edinburgh: Mosby.

Giddens, A. 1991. *Modernity and Self-Identity*. Palo Alto: Stanford University Press.

Kaptchuk, T. and Eisenberg, D. 1998. The persuasive appeal of alternative medicine. *Annals of Internal Medicine*, 129(12), 1061–5.

Lewith, G., Broomfield, J. and Prescott, P. 2002. Complementary cancer care in Southampton. *Complementary Therapies in Medicine*, 10, 100–106.

Low, J. 2004. Managing safety and risk. *Health*, 8(4), 445–63.

Lupton, D. and Tulloch, J. 2002. Risk is part of your life: Risk epistemologies among a group of Australians. *Sociology*, 36(2), 317–35.

McClean, S. 2005. 'The illness is part of the person': Discourses of blame, individual responsibility and individuation at a centre for spiritual healing in the north of England. *Sociology of Health and Illness*, 27(5), 628–48.

Morris, K., Johnston, N., Homer, L., and Walts, D. 2000. A comparison of complementary therapy use between breast cancer patients and patients with other primary tumor sites. *American Journal of Surgery*, 179(5), 407–11.

Rayner, L. and Easthope, G. 2001. Postmodern consumption and alternative medications. *Journal of Sociology*, 37(2), 157–76.

Siahpush, M. 1998. Postmodern values, dissatisfaction with conventional medicine and popularity of alternative therapies. *Journal of Sociology*, 34(1), 58–70.

Sointu, E. 2006. Recognition and the creation of wellbeing. *Sociology*, 40(3), 493–510.

Tovey, P., Atkin, K. and Milewa, T. 2001. The individual and primary care: Service user, reflexive choice maker and collective actor. *Critical Public Health*, 11(2), 153–66.

Chapter 9

Evidence-Based Paradigms and Contemporary Midwifery

Caroline Homer and Alex Broom

Introduction

Midwifery and maternity care are fields of community health where the use of evidence is, at best, contested and at worst highly divisive. The process of childbearing elicits strong opinions and views within Australian communities and in popular culture and there is often little evidence *per se* underpinning such debates. As a profession, midwifery is traditionally dominated by women and has strong links with feminist thought and community activism. At various points in time midwifery has had an antagonistic relationship with medicine, a profession historically dominated by men. This has resulted in a long period of inter-professional negotiation and conflict, although in more recent times there has been some convergence. Despite the increasing prominence and legitimacy of midwifery in maternity care, questions around what is safe, and who should provide care in the context of birthing, remains contentious. The evidence-based paradigm is influential in delineating what is safe and risky in the context of maternity care and thus shapes the relationship between midwifery and medicine.

The challenges that have occurred in development, use and interpretation of evidence in contemporary midwifery are exemplified in the practice of homebirth. In this chapter we investigate the politicising of evidence, focusing on how diverse philosophical and political perspectives have challenged the conventional evidence-based paradigm in the case of homebirth. Furthermore, through this analysis we examine the relationship between midwifery and evidence-based health care. Homebirth presents a contentious example of the problematic of evidence-based practice for midwifery. That is, how midwifery as a profession has attempted to negotiate the demands of integration (with obstetrics) *vis-à-vis* remaining distinct and retaining core values. Here we explore the politics of birthing in Australia the role of 'evidence' and evidence-based social movements therein.

The Development of an Evidence-Based Practice Approach in Maternity Care

Anecdotally, the development of evidence-based practice in maternity care occurred following the publication of Archie Cochrane's book *Effectiveness and*

Efficiency: Random Reflections on Health Services (Cochrane 1972). Cochrane, a British medical researcher, famously, awarded the "wooden spoon" to obstetrics. Cochrane argued that obstetrics had been particularly slow in its accumulation and application of valid evidence in clinical practice (Chalmers, Enkin and Keirse 1989: 3).

Following the publication of Cochrane's work in the early 1970s, obstetricians and midwives, and their respective organisations, began the process of assembling an international register of controlled trials in perinatal medicine. A team of obstetricians, midwives, epidemiologists and childbirth activists was led by Iain Chalmers of the Oxford Perinatal Epidemiology Unit. They conducted a search of medical databases, over 60 key journals and contacted researchers in the field in order to identify studies likely to provide the best evidence for evaluating the effectiveness of maternity care. The result was a seminal, two-volume, 1,500 page book entitled *Effective Care in Pregnancy and Childbirth* (Chalmers et al. 1989). Known informally as *Easy-Peesy*, this text led to a revolution in maternity care. For the first time maternity care providers had a resource based on systematic reviews of reliable research findings (from a biomedical perspective) that could assist women to make informed choices about their care. In order to make the findings more accessible for those involved in the care of childbearing women, *A Guide to Effective Care in Pregnancy and Childbirth* (Enkin et al. 2000) and more recently *A Cochrane Pocketbook: Pregnancy and Childbirth* (Hofmeyr et al. 2008) were published.

The inception and development of evidence-based medicine was inextricably tied to the critique and reconstruction of perinatal care internationally. The 1989 publication of *Effective Care in Pregnancy and Childbirth* represented an early attempt to address Cochrane's critiques and to summarise, by specialty or subspecialty, all relevant randomised controlled trials as a means to produce the best evidence (Cochrane 1979). This publication was received positively by the health care community and, as a result, the Director of Research and Development in the British National Health Service approved funding for Iain Chalmers to establish the Cochrane Centre (later renamed the Cochrane Collaboration) 'to facilitate the preparation of systematic reviews of randomised controlled trials of health care' (The Cochrane Collaboration 2010).

Evidence-Based Maternity Care: Fact or Fiction?

While the production of the systematic reviews on pregnancy and childbirth may have addressed the Cochrane critique, such resources were developed on the basis of a specific scientific understanding of what constitutes evidence. Given the diverse orientations of maternity care providers whose disciplines had different historical origins, the question of what constitutes legitimate knowledge remained key to the dynamics between professional groupings. The production of knowledge and evidence remains contested in many areas of maternity care.

Mary-Rose MacColl (2009) has highlighted this point, illustrating how a person's acceptance of 'evidence' depends more on personal beliefs than research findings. Her exploration of the politics behind birth in Australia illustrated that 'knowledge about many areas of maternity care remains contested, which means different experts have different opinions often supported by different elements of available research' (MacColl 2009: 37). Moreover, MacColl argues that so-called 'objective' reality tends to be rather elusive when mixed with the emotions of childbirth and the politics of evidence production.

Homebirth in Australia is a particularly political and contentious example of the complex interplay between the production and acceptance of evidence, and political influence. The emergent evidence surrounding the safety and benefits of homebirth is in flux and to date no randomised controlled trials have been undertaken or are likely to be undertaken in the foreseeable future (Keirse 2010). Thus, the evidence-base for or against homebirth remains highly contentious.

Homebirths account for a very small number of births in Australia. Only 0.3 per cent of all women who gave birth chose homebirth, according to recent national statistics (Laws, Li and Sullivan 2010). This is compared with 2.9 per cent in the same year in England and Wales (United Kingdom Office of National Statistics 2010) and 0.6 per cent in the United States in 2006 (MacDorman, Declercq, and Menacker 2011). A recent study from New Zealand reported that 11 per cent of healthy women choose to have a homebirth (Davis et al. 2011).

A recent national review of maternity services in Australia identified that homebirth was a sensitive and controversial issue (Commonwealth of Australia 2009). In particular, the review 'formed the view that the relationship between maternity health care professionals is not such as to support homebirth as a mainstream Commonwealth-funded option (at least in the short term)' (Commonwealth of Australia 2009: 20–21). The release of this Report in 2009 heralded the commencement of the most recent homebirth debate as will be detailed in this chapter.

The Homebirth Debate

Midwives have been attending women for many thousands of years, mostly at home. Some of the oldest records appear in the Bible where reference is made to a twin birth attended by a midwife (Genesis 38: 27–30). Clay tablets and papyrus records also describe female birth attendants and their practices around 1,700 BC (Dempsey 1949). At the beginning of the twentieth century approximately one percent of women in developed countries such as Britain and Australia gave birth in hospitals with the majority of women giving birth at home (Campbell and Macfarlane 1994). Towards the middle of the twentieth century, there was decline in the proportion of women giving birth at home as hospitals were seen as safer places in which to give birth (Keirse 2010). By the 1980s, only one percent of women gave birth at home in these two countries, making homebirth a minority activity (Campbell and Macfarlane 1994, Pilley Edwards 2005). This trend did not occur in all developed countries with the Netherlands being a notable exception (de Jong et al. 2009).

Arguments for and against homebirth exhibit a complex combination of embedded beliefs as to whether 'home is best' or 'hospital is safe' *and* clinical evidence of the risks related to a homebirth and the ability of the hospital to reduce this risk (van Weel, van der Velden and Lagro-Janssen 2009). The pro-homebirth lobby has argued that it is a women's choice where she gives birth and that homebirth, for appropriately selected women who have access to the care of a professional midwife, is safe. This position has been incorporated into health policy in countries where governments provide legislative and financial support for homebirth. For example, in the United Kingdom, the policy document for maternity services, *Maternity Matters*, pledged to provide high quality, safe and accessible maternity care through delivery of 'four national choice guarantees'. One of these four guarantees is the option for women to elect home birth (Department of Health 2007, RCOG and RCM 2007). In Australia, pro-homebirth groups have been increasingly politically active. This activism has included public demonstrations and a large public rally was held in the national capital Canberra in 2009. At this rally, pro-homebirth advocates called on the federal government to support a woman's right to choose a homebirth (Metherell 2009).

Those who argue that homebirth is an unsafe option posit that, no matter what safeguards are put in place, a birthing mother and her baby will never be as safe at home as they are in a hospital (Pesce 2010a). Media headlines in Australia such as 'A home birth is not a safe birth' have added to this argument (Devine 2009). The anti-homebirth lobby in many nations has explicitly perpetuated the notion that clinical surveillance and technological intervention is the safest option while birth at home is risky. From this perspective, the clinic rhetorically becomes the State's haven, protecting women from an unpredictable and precarious birthing process. In this sense, modern birthing is articulated as an ability to control and limit the risks of pre-modern non-clinical birthing practices; homebirth in many ways represents a return to an undesirable non-technological, precarious past.

Research illustrates that women choose homebirth for a wide variety of reasons. Some of these reasons include: wanting increased control over the birthing process; ensuring a continuity of care (birth at home and post-natal care at home); wishing to avoid the perceived unnecessary medical interventions; or, a broad dislike or fear of hospitals (Neuhaush et al. 2002, Viisainen 2001). As mentioned above, evidence around homebirth is highly contested, and, although large randomised controlled trials have *not* been undertaken, evidence from large descriptive studies that supports the safety of homebirth (de Jonge et al. 2009, Janssen et al. 2009, Johnson and Daviss 2005, Olsen and Jewell 1998). Studies in the USA (Johnson and Daviss 2005), Canada (Janssen et al. 2009) and the Netherlands (de Jonge et al. 2009), for example, involving more than 300,000 women, have shown that homebirth is safe for healthy women who do not have medical or obstetric risk factors, and where there are appropriate systems in place to provide emergency support and access to hospital care if required. These include effective communication between doctors and midwives at the local hospital, and the availability of ambulance services and a smooth transfer to hospital if required.

Despite the apparent descriptive (albeit not experimental/prospective) evidence of safety in the context of homebirth, in Australia there has been considerable negative publicity recently in the popular media (Devine 2009), heated debate amongst academics, maternity care providers, consumers and policy makers (Dahlen and Homer 2010, Ellwood 2008, Newman 2008). Medical colleges and associations in Australia and the United States strongly oppose homebirth. For example, The Royal Australian and New Zealand College of Obstetricians and Gynaecologists (RANZCOG), has always opposed homebirth and this has been reiterated in their recent guidelines which include blunt statements including 'RANZCOG does not endorse Home Birth' (RANZCOG 2008: 1); and 'Home Birth should not be offered as a "Model of Care"' (RANZCOG 2008: 4). The industrial union for doctors in Australia, the Australian Medical Association (AMA), continues to highlight their opposition to homebirth (Pesce 2010). Their Press Release in early 2010 stated 'The AMA does not support home birth because of the safety concerns for mother and baby' (AMA 2010). The American College of Obstetricians (ACOG) takes a similar line in their most recent statement, however, they do acknowledge that the problems with homebirth are related to inadequately trained attendants, women with serious high-risk medical conditions such as high blood pressure, breech births, or prior caesarean birth (ACOG 2011). Obstetrics often takes the view that childbirth is only normal in retrospect and so the capacity to deal with the unexpected consequences takes precedence (Kitzinger 2005, Silverton 1993). In an obstetric frame of reference, unexpected consequences can be better managed in a hospital situation.

The 'Politicking' of Homebirth in Australia

The national review of maternity services commissioned in 2008 by the Australian Federal Government added to the debate about homebirth, and resulted in the 'homebirth issue' becoming part of the formal political processes (Commonwealth of Australia 2009). There were more than 900 written submissions to the review – from consumers, professional organizations and individual practitioners. More than 60 per cent of the submissions were about homebirth – the vast majority from women who wanted access to homebirth. Of the professional submissions to the review, a number of midwifery organisations, including the peak professional group for midwives, the Australian College of Midwives, supported access to homebirth (Australian College of Midwives Queensland Branch 2008). Obstetric and medical organisations were strongly opposed (RANZCOG 2009). For example, in their submission, the Australian Medical Association stated that:

> There is strong evidence that we should not be considering publicly funded midwife led home birth. A 1998 Australian Study published in the BMJ showed

that in-home birthing by midwives is three times more likely to lead to perinatal mortality than conventional options even with the lowest risk pregnancies. (Australian Medical Association 2008: 10)

The AMA's statement provides an interesting example of the political use of 'evidence'. The Australian study that was cited by the AMA analysed data on planned homebirths that took place between 1985 and 1990 (Bastian, Keirse and Lancaster 1998). The births had been reported to Homebirth Australia, a national consumers' association that, at the time, kept a register of practitioners attending home births. The study was retrospective, included births by unregistered midwives, and used a number of different methods to collect the data including searching newsletters for death notices. The authors recognised these factors as limitations of the study and it seems likely that even they would not see it as providing 'strong evidence', as the AMA suggested it did. Despite the study having significant limitations in terms of methodology the Australian Medical Association was quite willing to accept it as evidence.

In fact, the situation is far more in favour of homebirth in terms of available evidence. The findings of Bastian, Keirse and Lancaster (1998) showed that homebirth was safe for healthy women who did not have medical or obstetric known risk factorsHigher rates of perinatal mortality (deaths in unborn and newborn babies) were to be found amongst women who did have risk factors (for example, twin pregnancy and babies in the breech position). The authors concluded that:

> While home birth for low risk women can compare favourably with hospital birth, high-risk home birth is inadvisable and experimental. (Bastian, Keirse and Lancaster 1998: 387)

Following the release of the Maternity Services Review in February 2009, the Federal Government supported many of the recommendations. The Federal budget in May of that year announced sweeping changes and reforms to maternity services including access for midwives to Commonwealth funding (Vernon 2009). Commonwealth funding for access to homebirth was not supported. The decision relating to homebirth was met with dismay by homebirth supporters and public rallies supporting homebirth were held in Canberra, Brisbane, Perth and Sydney as well as a number of regional areas (Dahlen et al. 2009).

In the Australian parliament, the issue of access to homebirth was fiercely debated. The parliamentary debate discussed homebirth using the submissions from women, midwives, obstetricians and other lobby groups. Arguments against homebirth, particularly from the Australian Medical Association included:

> The government was absolutely correct when it decided not to extend these bills to cover home births. The fundamental goal of maternity care must be a healthy mother and a healthy baby. ... It is not appropriate for the Commonwealth to

introduce payment and insurance arrangements that encourage or sanction activities that inherently carry more risk. (Chester 2009: 36)

Some others were more circumspect and suggested that all reasonable parties to such debate would rightly acknowledge that homebirthing is not an appropriate option for all women. One stated: '... I am here to defend the right of intelligent, informed Australian adults to have a choice – to be entitled to decide for themselves' (Dutton 2009: 27).

Through this political process, issues of illegality, insurance and professional control were played out with actual evidence, in any guise, playing a relatively minor role. The National Maternity Services Review, and reforms proposed in relation to national regulation of health professionals in Australia, came together in an unexpected and unplanned fashion. The national regulation of ten health disciplines had been on the political agenda for a number of years and was due to come into operation from mid 2010. One of the requirements of the new national regulation is that, in order to be registered, health professionals are required to hold professional indemnity insurance. Midwives in private practice who predominately provide homebirth services in Australia have been unable to access professional indemnity insurance since 2001 (Commonwealth of Australia 2009).

A Political Compromise or Political Silence ...

In late 2009, three Bills were presented to the Parliament of Australia. One was to support the inclusion of midwives under the Medicare Benefits Scheme and the Pharmaceutical Benefits Scheme and the other two were to enable the establishment of a professional indemnity scheme. These provisions would mean midwives could provide private care in the same way available to doctors. Following debate over the Maternity Services Review and considerable lobbying from both sides, the several key bills passed to the Upper House of the Australia Senate. The Senate referred the issue to the Community Affairs Legislation Committee for inquiry and report. Within a short period of time the committee had received nearly 2,000 submissions, primarily from midwives who provided homebirth services and parents who described their experiences with, and support for, homebirth (Moore et al. 2009).

The committee's conclusion was that the legislation did not take away any current rights and none of the Bills made homebirth unlawful and therefore they should be passed (Moore et al. 2009). A minority report from two opposition senators was published as part of the main report. This stated that 'expecting parents should have a right to choose where their child is born and that the Parliament must not allow the practice of home-birthing to go underground' (Moore et al. 2009: 21). They recommended a 'full inquiry into Home birthing in Australia' (Moore et al. 2009: 28). A Dissenting Report (Siewert 2009) was produced by the senator from the Green Party which was supportive of homebirth and recommended changes to enable homebirth to continue with access to professional indemnity insurance for midwives.

A political compromise saw midwifery care supported but not homebirth. Despite the plethora of evidence suggesting that women wanted access to homebirth the federal government did not support access to public funding for homebirth for Australian women. In March 2010, the Bills were passed in the Senate in what was lauded as '[a] landmark day for Australian nurses and midwives' (Roxon 2010). The media release was silent on the matter of homebirth indicating the political risk associated with public support or condemnation of homebirth.

Good and Bad News Stories

Negative portrayals of homebirth in the media have added to the aforementioned political and legislative challenges surrounding homebirth. Front page headlines like 'Four Dead in Homebirthing' (Lawrence and Dunlevy 2009) reported on the death of a homebirth activist's baby who was born at home unattended by a health professional. As a part of the moral framing of birth choices, Australian media attributed blame for the death on the homebirth rather than on the fact that it was an unattended birth (a birth without a midwife present). This particular case gained much exposure in the national media for the following three weeks, creating a moral panic around the dangers of homebirth (Dahlen 2010).

Some media analysis around this time was positive or more circumspect. For example, 'Home births just as safe' (Hall 2009) provided a balanced assessment of homebirth in *The Sydney Morning Herald*. 'Birth Rights' an article that appeared in *The Good Weekend*, the weekend magazine published by *The Sydney Morning Herald*, also provided a careful discussion of the evidence and politics surrounding homebirth in Australia (van Tiggelen 2009). This latter story presented the views of those for, and against, homebirth and in so doing highlighted the political landscape in which homebirth is seen in Australia. The president of the AMA, Andrew Pesce, was cited as 'blaming the more radical advocates of natural birth for demonising mainstream maternity services'. Hannah Dahlen from the Australian College of Midwives cautioned that 'birth should not be a political act' and raised concerns about the 'turf war against midwives' in the debate (van Tiggelen 2009). Place of birth thus became a political act and the media placed midwives and obstetricians in opposing sides of the so-called turf war. Once again, evidence for and against was used polemically and strategically to bolster a particular stakeholder position.

New Stories, Studies and Dilemmas

Six months after the homebirth activist story, homebirth was back in the Australia media, initially positively and then negatively. *The Sydney Morning Herald* ran a story titled 'Homebirth program that delivers' about the publicly-funded homebirth program established by St George Hospital in Sydney. The story was in response to a paper on the evaluation of the program released some weeks earlier (McMurtrie et al. 2009) and was accompanied with a photo of a happy mother and her baby who was born at home with midwives employed by the St George Hospital. A week later, the paper published a story titled 'Obstetricians urge caution on homebirths' which related to a press release and article published the day before by the *Medical Journal of Australia*. The aim of the paper was to establish baseline data prior to evaluating the impact of the homebirth policy introduced into South Australia (Kennare et al. 2010). The study compared the outcomes of over 250,000 planned hospital births in South Australia between 1991 and 2006 with those of 1,141 planned home births. This latter group was defined as any birth intended to occur at home at the time of antenatal booking and about 30 per cent of this group actually gave birth in hospital. There were nine perinatal deaths in the planned homebirth group and 2,440 deaths in the group with a planned hospital birth over the 16 years. Planned homebirths had a perinatal mortality rate similar to that for planned hospital births (7.9 for home birth compared with 8.2 for hospital birth per 1,000 births). There was a seven times higher risk of death of the baby during labour and a 27-times higher risk of death from asphyxia (lack of oxygen to the baby) during labour for home births as compared with hospital births. However, these figures must be attenuated against the small sample sizes in these sub-groups (two and three deaths respectively in the planned homebirth groups) that give rise to very wide confidence intervals indicating a high level of uncertainty in estimates. The authors themselves urged caution in the findings saying 'small numbers with large confidence intervals limit interpretation of these data' (Kennare et al. 2010: 79). These qualifications that inform a nuanced interpretation of the data were omitted in much of the resulting media and professional commentary that followed.

The Political Utility and Mis-Representation of 'Evidence'

The *Medical Journal of Australia* published an editorial to accompany the Kennare et al. (2010) paper and this, and much of the media in the next 48 hours, missed the subtlety of the caution. The editorial, written by the President of the AMA, was titled 'Planned home birth in Australia: politics or science?' (Pesce 2010a) and stated that 'given the accumulated evidence from Australia spanning 30 years, facilitating and funding home birth in an autonomous setting would be contrary to the principles of evidence-based health administration' (Pesce 2010a: 60). The accumulated evidence included the earlier study by Bastian et al. (1998) which, as was highlighted earlier, has been misquoted for more than decade in relation to the safety of homebirth for women without known risk factors. The press release focussed on high risk of death of the baby which occurred during the woman's labour but omitted the actual numbers of deaths (that is, two) or the uncertainty surrounding the estimates of increased risk (Sweet 2010).

A press release from the journal was picked up by almost every major media outlet in Australia with headlines such as 'Homebirth "more risky" than hospital delivery'. The electronic blogging media also ran with the story. One outlet, Crikey.com, published a series of posts critiquing the paper (Sweet 2010) with a response from the AMA titled 'The AMA says we are shooting the messenger re homebirth' (Pesce 2010b). The AMA President admitted that his editorial was primarily about the politics of homebirth. One of the authors of the original paper also posted a long and thoughtful commentary about the study, the Editorial, the critiques (one of which the present author has contributed to) and blogs.

The way the study was reported showed, yet again, the extent to which 'evidence' was appropriated within a political conflict, generating controversy in ways that would influence political decision regarding service delivery. The homebirth question was, and continues to be, a socio-political process in which evidence is posterior to politics. Melissa Sweet, a health journalist who coordinates health coverage for Crikey.com criticised the press release for fanning the fire of controversy and sensationalism (Sweet 2010). Most of the journalists admitted to Sweet that they had not read or even sourced the article highlighting the limitations of seeing the media as an accurate reporter of evidence.

Midwifery, Childbirth and Evidence

A key question is why birth, and particularly homebirth, became a political issue rather than an issue about health care provision. A popular explanation, feminist in orientation, is that homebirth takes us back to a birthing context of women supporting women at home; and women controlled the birth environment. Such ideas situate the debate around the idea that birth is socially produced and culturally located and it is only in the last 60 years that it has been medicalised within an acute hospital setting.

Historically, birth has taken place in domestic (women's) spaces; a domestic and maternal realm (Kitzinger 2005). Men were generally excluded from the room in which birth occurred at home (usually the bedroom). The ritual of childbirth, in such settings, was viewed as a critical process of bonding women (those giving birth and those assisting) with 'expert' knowledge was handed down in a matrilineal fashion, from mother to daughter. Traditional childbirth knowledge (or in today's terms, evidence) was based on feminine experience rather than texts and relied heavily on rituals to make birth safe that largely were driven by women (Kitzinger 2005).

From the sixteenth century until the middle of the twentieth century, most midwives were not formally educated, and as women, denied access to the increasing body of medical knowledge that was developing and taught within universities as part of medical education. An exception was to be found at the Hotel Dieu in Paris, a charitable monastic institution, founded in the sixteenth century in order to provide free birthing services to the poor as well as instruction for midwives (Leap 2001). By the eighteenth century this school was renowned throughout Europe. One of the Hotel Dieu's earliest scholars was Louise Bourgeois who educated midwives and became famous as the official royal midwife and writer of midwifery books. This work, with further enlarged editions in 1617, 1626, and 1634, contributed much to the advancement of French midwifery (Dunn 2004). The Hotel Dieu and the role models like Louise Bourgeois, provided those who attended with education and status as midwives, hence supporting the emergence of the profession of midwifery.

Increasingly though, the role of midwives was being taken over by male physicians. Known originally as the 'man midwife', the male birth attendant would eventually assume the title 'obstetrician' meaning 'to stand before' (Leap 2001: 495). The lucrative nature of attending the wealthy in childbirth attracted an increasing number of men into midwifery throughout seventeenth and eighteenth century Europe. The fashionable status symbol of employing men-midwives was boosted by the invention of the obstetric forceps and the gradual establishment of birth as a medical science. The convention of the time deemed that instruments could only be used by surgeons and only men could be surgeons (Leap 2001). This presented a severe threat to women who were employed as midwives. Educated midwives criticised the use of forceps by medical men seeing it as unnecessary intervention in what was a woman's domain. Elizabeth Cellier was an English political midwifery activist. In 1687, she proposed (unsuccessfully) establishing a corporation consisting of London midwives and using the fees to set up parish houses where any woman could give birth. The scheme included plans for a hospital and a college for instruction in midwifery similar to the Hotel Dieu (Leap 2001: 496).

A century later, Elizabeth Nihell, wrote the *Treatise on the Art of Midwifery, Setting Forth Various Abuses Therein, Especially as to the Practice with Instruments* (Nihell 1760). She had trained at the Hotel Dieu and practised in London as a midwife. She had a vested interest in trying to stem the rising tide of man-midwifery as not only were men entering the profession but it was being seen as fashionable, and by some, more safe to engage a male practitioner for childbirth (Cook and Collier Cook 2006). She was highly dismissive of male practitioners, admitting that while they were rare they were totally inferior to 'good' midwives, meaning, women (Nihell 1760: ix). She acknowledged that instruments were not within her sphere of practice (Nihell 1760: xiv) however, strongly argued that it was instruments used by men which had caused deaths and damage and was strident in her criticism:The surgeons, in [the] form of men-midwives, have been the death of more children with their speculum, their crochets, their extractors or forceps ... than they have preferred. If in killing the children, they have saved the lives of some mothers, they have hurt and damaged, not to say murdered, a number of others (Nihell 1760: 54).

Governing Midwives and the Consolidation of a 'Profession'

The First Midwives Act in England, *The Public General Acts 1902*, formalised the profession of midwifery. The Act aimed to secure the better training of midwives and to regulate their practice, within a sociohistorical context of unregulated and unsafe practices. Indeed, midwives included prostitutes who were reputedly paid in gin (Stevens 2002). As in other countries including Australia, legislation would also ensure that the regulation of midwifery practice and education would support the development of a respected profession (Barclay 2008).

With the regulation of midwifery co-evolving with its professionalising within educational institutions, medicine and midwifery have co-existed, albeit developing in parallel, for some centuries; however it continues to be a contested relationship with both groups claiming to practice using an evidence-based approach (Fahy 2007). The perceived status of both medicine and midwives has added complexity to the authority of evidence with class and gender having been seen as mechanisms which supported the differentiation between medical doctors and their competitors including midwives (Willis 1983). In the last 100 years, the independent status of the midwife has significantly diminished as has home birth as a viable option to hospital birth. Birth for the majority women in Australia, Britain and other developed nations now takes place in institutions which rely on highly specialised staff and complex technical equipment and essentially supports a medical dominance (Barclay 2008). Willis, a labour sociologist has argued that the medical profession achieved its dominance over the Australian health system and has defended this dominance against other health care occupations since (Willis 1983).

The question of professional dominance in childbirth has led to heated debate in the media and the academic and professional literature that often positions midwives and doctors as opposing forces. The historical tensions and ideological differences between medicine and midwifery are often seen as being so great that they need 'managing' rather attempting to 'overcome' (Dahlen 2006). Indeed, much of the tension is situated within economic and politics interests and influence. The expansion of midwifery care in the twentieth and now twenty-first centuries represents a significant threat to doctors' incomes, power base and a deeply held faith in the biomedical model. Yet, there is little public acknowledgement of the economic and political control of maternity care, Rather, as Dahlen writes in reference to the obstetrics community, 'they argue safety and instill fear' (Dahlen 2006: 6).

The parallel development of medicine and midwifery has ensured the persistence of key, historically rooted differences in practice. Homebirth highlights a fundamental difference in the management of childbirth to that of medical approaches, most notably its 'non-technological' approach. In contrast, childbirth takes place with as little external intervention as possible the woman's body is conceptualised as having the capacity to give birth without extraneous interference. A technological view is illustrated in most contemporary hospitals, where technology, even if not required or used must be available (Davis-Floyd 2001). Davis-Floyd, a cultural anthropologist, believes the impetus to improve on 'nature' through technology occurs as an attempt to free us from the limitations of nature. The technocratic imperative means freedom from the limitations of birth through obstetrics (Davis-Floyd 1994). In this paradigm, there is a desire and need to control 'nature'. Davis-Floyd describes how birth has been deconstructed and technocricised under this paradigm (Davis-Floyd 1994). Birth is feared as chaotic, uncontrollable, and therefore dangerous. Thus birth is considered to be improved through technology using interventions like electronic monitoring and medications, or a baby rescued with even more technology (episiotomy, forceps or caesarean section). Homebirth is the antithesis of these processes of improvement or rescue.

Evidence and Midwifery as Social Movements

This final section on the politics of homebirth examines different views of the nature of evidence and the challenge of obtaining 'acceptable' evidence. Homebirth is a difficult area in terms of the pursuit of evidence that meets the biomedical gold standard for interventions – the randomised controlled trial (Timmermans and Berg 2003). While one way of improving the evidence, and potentially reducing the contested nature of the evidence, would be evaluate to homebirth in a randomised controlled trial, this is not likely to be feasible in Australia or in many other similar countries. In many respects EBM as a social movement was premised on a desire to bring to an end the uncertainty of 'evidence' in and around birthing. Yet, as Oakley (1992) identified fairly early on in the development of EBM, the RCT is of limited use in the context of researching birthing preferences and values or the risks of particularly models. Murray Enkin, the co-author of the original *Effective Care in Pregnancy and Childbirth* has acknowledged that many things that are relevant to questions of childbirth are not encompassed within the bounds of inquiry that evidence-based approaches can illuminate (Jadad and Enkin 2007). Moreover, the stratification of women's preferences in regards to childbirth correlate with factors that influence the research that may take place. Thus, as Fahy (2006), a midwife, has suggested:

> [A]nother limitation of evidence-based medicine is that the conduct of a clinical RCT requires support from all relevant clinicians and managers. This means that in maternity care, those with the funding and authority are able to conduct RCTs, whilst those with less power and funding are much more likely to be impeded by these barriers. (Fahy 2006: 2)

By those with less power, Fahy refers to midwives. Another challenge is the defining of outcome measures, a necessity in a trial. From whose perspective should this take place – the women, her family, the doctors or midwife or the organisation? The definition of an optimal outcome may be different within and between these groups and the notion of what constitutes risk and how this is interpreted will vary. For example, the value of psychological health over physical health could be privileged differently. The time period in which pregnancy and birth occur also creates difficulties in terms of recruitment to trials (Fahy and Tracy 2006). For example, a trial about the safety of a birth centre or a homebirth model of care would require recruitment of women early in pregnancy as they would require the intervention over the course of the pregnancy. The planned place of birth may change through the pregnancy as the clinical situation changes (for example if complications develop) however, women would be analysed in the group to which they were allocated even if this was not what ultimately occurred.

Problems in the production of a biomedical knowledge base for homebirth have been shown in various studies internationally. In the Netherlands, women refused participate in an RCT because they had already chosen their place of birth early in pregnancy (Hendrix et al. 2009). In the mid 1990s, a feasibility RCT of homebirth in the UK only managed to randomise 11 of 71 (16 per cent) of women (Dowswell et al. 1996). Some of the 60 women who declined to participate expressed themselves strongly, declaring that there was no chance or no way that they would take part in such a trial. Birth is such a cataclysmic event that finding women and families who are prepared to let the play of chance determine their choice of place of birth is unlikely.

Another challenge in conducting an RCT of the safety of home birth is the size of the study that would be required. If perinatal mortality was to be the primary outcome, then very large numbers of women would need to be recruited given that perinatal mortality is relatively rare among low risk women.

Homebirth and Evidence: The Controversy Continues

Given design limitations in the production of evidence for homebirth, systematic review and synthesis of all evidence available would seem a logical way forward for guiding policy and practice. However, even the process of systematic review is fraught with political and stakeholder challenges. For example, in 2010 the *American Journal of Obstetrics and Gynecology (AJOG)* published a systematic review on maternal and newborn safety of planned home versus planned hospital birth (Wax et al. 2010). Their study concluded that less medical intervention during planned home birth is associated with a tripling of the neonatal mortality rate. The percentage rose from 0.04 per cent for a hospital birth to 0.15 per cent for a home birth but the risks for perinatal mortality (death of the baby up to a week after birth) were similar for home and hospital birth. Home birth was also found to reduce the risk of interventions for the mother (for example, episiotomies, epidurals, caesareans). The systematic review has been thoroughly criticised in the academic literature and popular media with a number of subsequent commentaries and letters published (Keirse 2010).

The prestigious medical journal *The Lancet* drew attention to the Wax et al. study with an Editorial titled 'Homebirth – Proceed with caution' (*The Lancet* 2010: 303) including statements like 'women do not have the right to put their baby at risk.' The journal received, in their own words, a tidal wave of criticism (Horton 2010). Many of the letters received by *The Lancet* highlighted the deficiencies in *The AJOG* systematic review including the selective inclusion of studies to calculate mortality rates and the lack of critique of methodological quality of the original studies (Gyte, Dodwell and MacFarlane 2010). Other criticisms centred on paternalism (Bewley, Newburn and Sandall 2010) and the rights versus interests question with mothers being reduced to a mere factor in the perinatal decision process. This, according to many commentators, is directly deleterious to women's rights to self-determination (Kingmaa 2010: 1298).

Since *The AJOG* publication, a number of prominent researchers including some of those who were authors of papers included in the systematic review, have written to the editors of *AJOG* asking that the paper be retracted arguing that the article is 'deeply flawed'. Their nine-page letter pointed to mistakes in definitions, numerical errors, selective and mistaken inclusion and exclusion of studies, conflation of association and causation, and additional statistical problems. These authors asked that the editors of *AJOG* act with 'urgency and concern' to address the 'insupportable conclusion' of the article. In a similar way to the Australian study discussed previously in this chapter, *The AJOG* had also issued what was seen as a highly misleading press release to advertise the paper and they were requested to issue a press release announcing the retraction (Horton 2010). No retraction or comment from *The AJOG* has been made in response to this call.

Notwithstanding the major criticisms of the Wax et al. (2010) study, these and other studies highlighted the fraught area of the interpretation of risk especially in the context of homebirth. The question raised is would a risk of 0.15 per cent or 0.04 per cent deter women from having a homebirth and how does a person (clinician or pregnant woman) make judgments about risks at that level? Kotaska, a Canadian obstetrician has hypothesised that risk in maternity care has led to intervention through what he coined as the '1:1000 club' (Dahlen 2010). The increased risk of stillbirth late in pregnancy and the risk of perinatal death as a result of a vaginal breech birth are both good examples. That is, the emphasis is firmly placed on the one adverse event and thus focusing on the potential negative outcome as the only certainty highlighted by the evidence. There is often not an acknowledgment that such statistics also indicate that 999 times out of 1000 the outcome will be positive (Dahlen 2010).

Conclusion

This chapter has sketched the historic antecedents influencing the production of contemporary knowledge in the context of childbirth. A historical parallelism in the development of obstetrics and midwifery, in combination with issues of gender and class, has been partly responsible for the dearth of an evidentiary basis with regards to homebirth that is satisfactory to key authority figures in the medical profession and their supportive institutions. Furthermore, highly politicised contemporary debates continue to feed the division between pro and anti-homebirth stakeholders, hampering the development of syncretic approaches that may overcome the antagonist duality that has developed.

Evidence is not a neutral concept, and the production of evidence is politically laden with various groups standing to gain or lose from the adoption of their particular 'take' on evidence (Walsh 2007). The current 'evidence' available in and around maternity care is similarly contested with the range of experts having different views often based on competing studies (MacColl 2009). Evidence and research about birth, especially homebirth, is often emotionally charged and laden with politics and notions of power including who has the right to make such a choice. Evidence-based medicine was always intended to incorporate the needs and wants of the 'patient' (Sackett et al. 1997) but this has not always been the case in practice. It can, and has been used, as a blunt instrument to 'bludgeon the other side in the birth wars' (MacColl 2009: 40).

While some women do choose to give birth at home, politicising around this issue will no doubt continue making it difficult for many women to utilise this birthing option (and gain State funding to support it). Homebirth will continue to be a key site of struggle around risk and uncertainty, with EBCH devices and technologies utilised to justify *and* critique its representations within the popular media and academic literature.

Biomedical 'evidence' has strategically been used to demonise *and* validate homebirth with evidence deployed for professional and political interests rather than the pursuit of objectivity. It remains the case that homebirth is largely not a debate about evidence; it is more about a struggle over control of birthing, women's bodies, political power and control within the health system. A balance is now required between evidence and politics that does not forget that birth is a significant life experience for women, their partners and families.

References

American College of Obstetricians and Gynecologists. 2011. *The American College of Obstetricians and Gynaecologists Issues Opinion on Planned Home Births*. [Online]. Available at: http://www.acog.org/from_home/publications/press_releases/nr01-20-11.cfm [accessed: 10 April 2011].

Australian College of Midwives Queensland Branch. 2008. *Submission 663 – Australian College of Midwives Queensland Branch*. [Online]. Available at: http://www.health.gov.au/internet/main/publishing.nsf/Content/maternity servicesreview-663 [accessed: 16 March 2010]

Australian Medical Association (AMA). 2008. *AMA Submission to the Maternity Services Review*. [Online]. Available at: http://www.ama.com.au/node/4225 [accessed: 16 March 2010].

Australian Medical Association (AMA). 2010. *New Study Confirms High Risks of Home Births*. [Online]. Available at: http://ama.com.au/node/5273 [accessed: 12 April 2011].

Barclay, L. 2008. A feminist history of Australian midwifery from colonisation until the 1980s. *Women and Birth*, 21(1), 3–8.

Bastian, H., Keirse, M. and Lancaster, P. 1998. Perinatal death associated with planned home birth in Australia: Population based study. *British Medical Journal*, 317(7155), 384–8.

Bewley, S., Newburn, M. and Sandall, J. 2010. Editorials about home birth – Proceed with caution. *The Lancet*, 376(9749), 303

Campbell, R. and Macfarlane, A. 1994. *Where to be Born? The Debate and the Evidence*. Oxford: National Perinatal Epidemiology Unit.

Chalmers, I., Enkin, M. and Keirse, M.J.N.C. 1989. *Effective Care in Pregnancy and Childbirth*. Oxford: Oxford University Press.

Cochrane, A. 1972. *Effectiveness and Efficiency: Random Reflections on Health*. London: Nuffield Provincial Hospitals Trust.

Cochrane, A. 1979. 1931–1971: A critical review, with particular reference to the medical profession, in *Medicines for the Year 2000*. London: Office of Health Economics, 1–11.

Commonwealth of Australia. 2009. *Improving Maternity Services in Australia: Report of the Maternity Services Review*. Canberra: Commonwealth of Australia.

Cook, J. and Cook B. 2006. *Man-Midwife, Male Feminist: The Life and Times of George Macaulay, M.D., Ph.D. (1716–1766)*. Michigan: The Scholarly Publishing Office.

Dahlen, H. 2006. Midwifery: 'At the edge of history'. *Women and Birth,* 19(1), 3–10.

Dahlen, H. 2010. Undone by fear? Deluded by trust? *Midwifery*, 26(2), 156–62.

Dahlen, H. and Homer, C. 2010. *More Critique of the Homebirth Study and its Reporting by the Media*. [Online]. Available at: http://blogs.crikey.com.au/croakey/2010/01/20/more-critique-of-the-homebirth-study-and-its-reporting-by-the-media/ [accessed: 15 February 2010].

Dahlen, H., Vernon, B. and Wilkes, L 2009. Proposed amendments to the maternity reform bills. *Australian Midwifery News*, Summer, 4–6.

Davis, D., Baddock, S., Pairman, S., Hunter, M., Benn, C., Wilson, D., Dixon, L. and Herbison, P. 2011. Planned place of birth in New Zealand: Does it affect mode of birth and intervention rates among low-risk women? *Birth*, 38 (1), 1-9. DOI: 10.1111/j.1523-536X.2010.00458.

Davis-Floyd, R. 1994. Culture and birth: The technocratic imperative. *International Journal of Childbirth Education*, 9(2), 6–7.

Davis-Floyd, R. 2001. The technocratic, humanistic, and holistic paradigms of childbirth. *International Journal of Gynecology and Obstetrics*, 75(1), S5–S23.

de Jonge, A., van der Goes, B., Ravelli, A., Amelink-Verburg, M., Mol, B., Nijhuis, J., Gravenhorst, J. and Buitendijk, S. 2009. Perinatal mortality and morbidity in a nationwide cohort of 529,688 low-risk planned home and hospital births.

BJOG: An International Journal of Obstetrics and Gynaecology, 116(9), 1177–84.

Dempsey, A. 1949. A brief survey of early midwifery practice. *The Ulster Medical Journal*, XVIII(2), 109–15.

Department of Health. 2007. *Maternity Matters: Choice, Access and Continuity of Care in a Safe Service*. London: Department and Health.

Devine, M. 2009. A home birth is not a safe birth. *Sydney Morning Herald*. 9 April. [Online]. Available at: http://www.smh.com.au/lifestyle/lifematters/a-home-birth-is-not-a-safe-birth-20090408-a0s3.html [accessed: 11 April 2011].

Dickens, C. 1844. *The Life and Adventures of Martin Chuzzlewit*. London: Chapman and Hall.

Dowswell, T., Thornton, J., Hewison, J., Lilford, R., Raisler, J., Macfarlane, A., Young, G., Newburn, R., Dodds, R. and Settatree, R. 1996. Should there be a trial of home versus hospital delivery in the United Kingdom? *British Medical Journal*, 312(7033), 753–7.

Ellwood, D. 2008. The debate about place of birth. *Australian and New Zealand Journal of Obstetrics and Gynaecology*, 48(5), 449.

Enkin, M., Keirse, M., Neilson, J., Crowther, C., Duley, L., Hodnett, E. and Hofmeyr, J. 2000. *A Guide to Effective Care in Pregnancy and Childbirth*. Oxford: Oxford University Press.

Fahy, K. 2007. An Australian history of the subordination of midwifery. *Women and Birth*, 20(1), 25–9.

Fahy, K. and Tracy, S. 2006. Birth centre trials are unreliable. *Medical Journal of Australia*, 185(7), 407.

Gelbart, N. 1998. *The King's Midwife: A History and Mystery of Madame du Coudray*. Berkeley and Los Angeles: University of California Press.

Gyte, G., Dodwell, M. and MacFarlane, A. 2010. Editorials about home birth – Proceed with caution. *The Lancet*, 376(9749), 1297.

Hall, L. 2009. Midwife home birth as safe as hospital. *Sydney Morning Herald*, April 17. [Online]. Available at: http://www.smh.com.au/lifestyle/lifematters/midwife-home-birth-as-safe-as-hospital-says-study-20090416-a8wu.html [accessed: 12 April 2011].

Health Legislation Amendment (Midwives and Nurse Practitioners) Bill 2010. (Act no. 29) Canberra: Commonwealth of Australia.

Hemminki, E. and Merilainen, J. 1996. Long-term effects of cesarean sections: Ectopic pregnancies and placental problems. *American Journal of Obstetrics and Gynecology*, 174(5), 1569–74.

Hendrix, M., Van Horck, M., Moreta, D., Nieman, F., Nieuwenhuijze, M., Severens, J. and Nijhuis, J. 2009. Why women do not accept randomisation for place of birth: Feasibility of a RCT in the Netherlands. *BJOG: An International Journal of Obstetrics and Gynaecology*, 116(4), 537–44.

The Public General Acts Passed in the Second Year of the Reign of His Majesty King Edward the Seventh. The Midwives Act 1902. London: Printed for His Majesty's Stationery Office.

Hofmeyr, G., Neilsen, J., Alfirevic, Z., Crowther, C., Duley, L., Gulmezoglu, M., Gyte, G. and Hodnett, E. 2008. *A Cochrane Pocketbook: Pregnancy and Childbirth*. Chichester: The Cochrane Collaboration and John Wiley and Sons Ltd.

Horton, R. 2010. Urgency and concern about home births. *The Lancet*, 376(9755), 1812.

Jadad, A.R. and Enkin, M.W. 2007. *Randomized Controlled Trials: Questions, Answers and Musings*. 2nd Edition. Oxford: Blackwell Publishing.

Janssen, P., Saxell, L., Page, L., Klein, M., Liston, R. and Lee, S. 2009. Outcomes of planned home birth with registered midwife versus planned hospital birth with midwife or physician. *Canadian Medical Association Journal*, 181(6–7), 377–83.

Johnson, K. and Daviss, B. 2005. Outcomes of planned home births with certified professional midwives: Large prospective study in North America. *British Medical Journal*, 330(7505), 1416–22.

Keirse, M. 2010. Home birth: Gone away, gone astray, and here to stay. *Birth*, 37(4), 341–6.

Kennare, R., Keirse, M., Tucker, G. and Chan, A. 2010. Planned home and hospital births in South Australia, 1991–2006: Differences in outcomes. *Medical Journal of Australia*, 192(2), 76–80.

Kingmaa, E. 2010. Editorials about home birth – Proceed with caution. *The Lancet*, 376(9749), 1298.

Kitzinger, S. 2005. *The Politics of Birth*. Edinburgh: Elsevier Limited.

Lawrence, K. and Dunlevy, S. 2009. Four dead in homebirthing. *The Daily Telegraph*, April 6. [Online]. Available at: http://www.dailytelegraph.com.au/news/four-dead-in-home-birthing-including-joyous-birth-advocate/story-e6freuy9-1225697745818 [accessed: 11 April 2011].

Laws, P., Li, Z. and Sullivan, E. 2010. *Australia's Mothers and Babies 2008*. Canberra, Australian Institute of Health and Welfare, National Perinatal Statistics Unit.

Leap, N. 2001. Midwifery, in *The Oxford Illustrated Companion to Medicine*, edited by L. Lock, J. Last and G. Dunea. Oxford: Oxford University Press, 493–8.

MacColl, M. 2009. *The Birth Wars*. St Lucia: University of Queensland Press.

MacDorman, M., Declercq, E., Menacker, F. and Malloy, M.H. 2006. Infant and neonatal mortality for primary cesarean and vaginal births to women with 'no indicated risk', United States, 1998–2001 birth cohorts. *Birth*, 33(3), 175–82.

MacDorman, M.F., Declercq, E. and Menacker, F. 2011. Trends and characteristics of home births in the United States by race and ethnicity, 1990–2006. *Birth*, 38(1), 17–23.

McMurtrie, J., Catling-Paul, C., Teate, A., Caplice, S., Chapman, M. and Homer, C.S.E. 2009. The St. George Homebirth Program: An evaluation of the first 100 booked women. *Australian and New Zealand Journal of Obstetrics and Gynaecology*, 49(6), 631–6.

Metherell, M. 2009. "Mother of all rallies' for home birth. *Sydney Morning Herald.* 8 September. [Online]. Available at: http://www.smh.com.au/lifestyle/wellbeing/mother-of-all-rallies-for-home-birth-20090907-feel.html [accessed: 11 April 2011].

Moore, C., Siewert, R., Adams, J., Boyce, S., Brown, C., Furner, C., Fielding, S. 2009. Community Affairs Legislation Committee Health Legislation Amendment (Midwives and Nurse Practitioners) Bill 2009 and two related Bills [Provisions]. Canberra, Commonwealth of Australia. [Online]. Available at: http://www.aph.gov.au/senate/committee/clac_ctte/health_leg_midwives_nurse_practitioners_09_nov09/report/index.htm [accessed: 12 April 2011].

Neuhaus, W., Piroth, C., Kiencke, P., Göhring, U. and Mallman, P. 2002. A psychosocial analysis of women planning birth outside hospital. *Journal of Obstetrics Gynaecology*, 22(2), 143–9.

Newman, L. 2008. Why planned attended homebirth should be more widely supported in Australia. *Australian and New Zealand Journal of Obstetrics and Gynaecology*, 48(5), 450–53.

Nihell, E. 1760. *A Treatise on the Art of Midwifery, Setting Forth Various Abuses Therein, Especially as to the Practice with Instruments*. London: Printed for A. Morley.

Oakley, A. 1992. Getting at the oyster: One of the many lessons from the Social Support and Pregnancy Outcome Study, in *Women's Health Matters*, edited by H. Roberts. London: Routledge and Kegan Paul, 11–32.

Olsen, O. and Jewell, D. 1998. Home versus hospital birth. *Cochrane Database of Systematic Reviews* [Online]. Issue 3. Art. No.: CD000352. DOI: 10.1002/14651858.CD000352 [accessed: 11 April 2011].

Pesce, A. 2010a. Planned home birth in Australia: Politics or science? *Medical Journal of Australia*, 192(2), 60.

Pesce, A. 2010b. The AMA says we are 'shooting the messenger' re homebirth critique. 21 January. [Online]. Available at: http://blogs.crikey.com.au/croakey/2010/01/21/the-ama-says-we-are-shooting-the-messenger-re-homebirth-critique/ [accessed: 11 April 2011].

Pilley Edwards, N. 2005. *Birthing Autonomy: Women's Experiences of Planning Home Births*. Abingdon: Routledge.

Royal Australian and New Zealand College of Obstetricians and Gynaecologists. 2009. *College Statement: Homebirths*. Melbourne: Royal Australian and New Zealand College of Obstetricians and Gynaecologists. [Online]. Available at: http://www.ranzcog.edu.au/publications/statements/C-obs2.pdf [accessed: 11 April 2011].

Royal Australian and New Zealand College of Obstetricians and Gynaecologists. 2009. *Submission to the Maternity Services Review (Submission 400)*. [Online]. Available at: http://www.health.gov.au/internet/main/publishing.nsf/Content/maternityservicesreview-400/$FILE/400_The%20Royal%20Australian%20and%20New%20Zealand%20College%20of%20Obstetricians%20and%20Gynaecologists.pdf [accessed: 16 March 2010].

Royal College of Obstetricians and Gynaecologists and the Royal College of Midwives (RCOG and RCM). 2007. *Homebirth: Joint statement No.2, April 2007*. [Online]. Available at: http://www.rcmnormalbirth.net/webfiles/Statement/Home%20Births_Joint%20Statement.pdf [accessed: 17 February 2010].

Roxon, N. 2010. *A Landmark Day for Australian Nurses and Midwives*. 16 March. [Online]. Available at: http://www.health.gov.au/internet/ministers/publishing.nsf/Content/BC67CE5F41D17836CA2576E80012EEEB/$File/nr050.pdf [accessed: 19 May 2010].

Sackett, D., Richardson, W., Rosenberg,W. and Hayes,R. 1997. *Evidence-based Medicine: How to Practice and Teach EBM*. Sydney: Churchill Livingstone.

Siewert, R. 2009. Dissenting Report. [Online]. Available at: http://www.aph.gov.au/senate/committee/clac_ctte/health_leg_midwives_nurse_practitioners_09/report/d02.htm [accessed: 12 April 2011].

Silverton, L. 1993. *The Art and Science of Midwifery*. Hertfordshire: Prentice Hall International.

Stevens, R. 2002. The Midwives Act 1902: An historical landmark. *Midwives Magazine*. [Online]. Available at: http://www.rcm.org.uk/midwives/features/the-midwives-act-1902-an-historical-landmark [accessed: 20 January 2011].

Sweet, M. 2010. More on the homebirth study fracas – Some indepth reading. 2 March. [Online]. Available at: http://blogs.crikey.com.au/croakey/2010/03/02/more-on-the-homebirth-study-fracas-some-indepth-reading/ [accessed: 11 April 2011].

Sweet, M. 2010. Science, politics, and headlines in the home birth war. *British Medical Journal*, 340, c826.

The Cochrane Collaboration. 2010. *History: The Cochrane Collaboration*. [Online]. Available at: http://www.cochrane.org/about-us/history [accessed: 23 January 2011].

The Lancet. 2010. Home birth – Proceed with caution. *The Lancet*, 376(9738), 303.

Timmermans, S. and Berg, M. 2003. *The Gold Standard: The Challenge of Evidence-Based Medicine and Standardization in Health Care*. Philadelphia: Temple.

Van Blarcom, C. 1913. *The Midwife in England, Being a Study in England of the Working of the English Midwives Act of 1902*. New York City: 130 East 22nd Street.

van Tiggelen, J. 2009. Birth rights. *The Good Weekend*. 5 September, 14–19.

van Weel, C., van der Velden, K. and Lagro-Janssen, T. 2009. Home births revisited: The continuing search for better evidence. *BJOG: An International Journal of Obstetrics and Gynaeocology*, 116(9), 1149–50.

Vernon, B. 2009. Roxon champions maternity reform: Medicare for midwives. *Australian Midwifery News*, Winter, 4–5.

Viisainen, K. 2001. Negotiating control and meaning: Home birth as a self-constructed choice in Finland. *Social Science and Medicine*, 52(7), 1109–21.

Walsh, D. 2007. *Evidence-based Care for Normal Labour and Birth: A Guide for Midwives.* London: Routledge.

United Kingdom Office of National Statistics. 2010. *Live Births in England and Wales by Characteristics of Birth.* [Online]. Available at: http://www.statistics.gov.uk/pdfdir/birth1110.pdf [accessed: 12 April 2011].

Wax, J., Lucas, F., Lamont, M., Pinette, M., Cartin, A. and Blackstone, J. 2010. Maternal and newborn outcomes in planned homebirth vs planned hospital births: A meta-analysis. *American Journal of Obstetrics and Gynecology*, 203(243), e1–8.

Willis, E. 1983. *Medical Dominance: The Division of Labour in Australian Health Care.* Sydney: Allen and Unwin.

Yang, Q., Wen, S., Oppenheimer, L., Chen, X., Black, D., Gao, J. and Walker, M. 2007. Association of caesarean delivery for first birth with placenta praevia and placental abruption in second pregnancy. *BJOG: An International Journal of Obstetrics and Gynaecology*, 114(5), 609–13.

Chapter 10
Evidence-Based Healthcare:
The Future Research Agenda

Anne-Grete Sandaunet and Evan Willis

Introduction

In this last chapter, the aim is to outline some crucial issues for future research on evidence-based health care in the social sciences. Consistent with the approach taken in this book, the phenomenon of evidence-based medicine (EBM) is analysed in social science terms. EBM is approached as a social movement with widespread significance in contemporary health care (Banta 2003, Behague et al. 2009, Broom, Adams and Tovey 2009, Pope 2003, Timmermans and Almeling 2009).

The debate on EBM including the emergence of evidence-based health care has been characterised and framed by polarised positions (Timmermans and Mauck 2005). EBM is considered a powerful problem solver by its proponents and by its critics as creating 'cookbook medicine'. On the whole, social scientists have tended to place themselves among the more critical voices, warning of the negative consequences of EBM implementation. This has included highlighting such aspects as the corrosion of individual medical judgement (Rodwin 2001) and patients mere passive recipients of expertise (Frankford 1994). A call to move on from these concerns and a suggestion of new avenues for research was provided by Mykhalovskiy and Weir (2004) and has been taken further by Timmermans and Mauck (2005) as well as Broom, Adams and Tovey (2009). These contributions recommend that futuresocial science research on EBM be empirically grounded (e.g. Mykhalovskiy and Weir 2004), looking beyond the predicated success of EBM (e.g. Timmermans and Mauck 2005). The importance of taking account of local and situational factors has been emphasised in particular, and the question of how such factors interact with the attempted standardisation of health care that many see as the core element of EBM.

This chapter supports this call for a broader approach within social science research on EBM and EBHC more broadly. The argument proposed is that the implementation of EBM-type models has turned out to be a bumpier road than the straightforward process that was assumed to be a decade ago. The key components of our argument are outlined in the first part of this chapter. While initially paying attention to clinical contexts, the main emphasis here is placed on EBM as manifest in health-related political decision making. Based on this outline, the latter part of the chapter examines some implications for further research.

EBM on a 'Bumpier' Road than First Assumed?

In tracing the emergence of EBM, one common approach is to explore the use and production of clinical practical guidelines (CPG) (Knaapen et al. 2010, Timmermans and Berg 2003). In the classic definition by Field and Lohr (1990:18), CPGs are defined as 'systematically developed statements to assist practitioner and patient decisions about appropriate health care for specific clinical circumstances'. For one of the founders of 'first wave' EBM, David Sackett (Sackett et al. 1996), CPG's are considered crucial for the delivery of best practice in health care. CPG's are constructed for, and used in, clinical contexts which include not only medical treatment, but also therapeutic, rehabilitative and preventive health care delivery (Field and Lohr 1990).

Previous medical and social science research has explored the use and production of CPGs, as the 'key component' of EBM (Knaapen et al. 2010). Regarding the use of guidelines, it has, for example, been demonstrated that few CPGs lead to actual changes in provider behaviour (Timmermans and Mauck 2005) and that their impact on clinical practice is highly variable (Carlsen, Glenton and Pope 2007). A range of barriers to evidence-based practice and successful guideline implementation have also been identified (Carlsen, Glenton and Pope 2007, McKinlay et al. 2004). These include clinician resistance to managerial culture (or deskilling) and the lack of applicability of a CPG for the individual patient. Carlsen, Glenton and Pope (2007) in their study found that GPs' reasons for not following guidelines differed according to whether the guideline in question was prescriptive, in that it encouraged a certain type of behaviour or treatment, or proscriptive, in that it discouraged certain treatments or behaviours. That is, such things as tone, wording and the perception of 'being managed' make a difference in the uptake of evidence guidelines. Adding weight to the complex implementation processes of EBM in clinical contexts, Broom, Adams and Tovey (2009) illustrate significant variations in perception of EBM between oncology sub-specialities in Australia.

Another challenging process for EBM is the character of political decision making and its influence on service delivery. During the last decade, requirements of a 'post-ideological' politics that is based on scientific facts have entered a number of non-clinical public policy areas (Behague et al. 2009, May 2006). Within the health care area, political decisions are intended to be made in reference to evidence-based practice. Certain evaluation tools, such as Health Technology Assessment (HTA) or Comparative Effectiveness Research (CER), have been developed to make EBM-type models a suitable political decision making tool. This has meant that cost-effectiveness, in addition to social and ethical issues, is intended to be taken into consideration (Banta 2003, Chalkidou et al. 2009). The scope of interventions that can be assessed by these evaluation tools is broad, including both counselling services and patient information websites (Banta 2003, Chalkidou et al. 2009). CER is a term which has developed in the US, but several other countries use CER in their efforts to determine aspects of health policy (Chalkidou et al. 2009, Coulter 2011). CER is an improved evaluative tool for evidence-based policy making and gained particular attention in the US in 2009 when the budget for this research was considerably increased (Coulter 2011).

It is within this context that contemporary political decision making in health care takes place, and which is here argued to constitute an important area for future social science research on EBM. Three examples are presented below in order to outline the argument of a bumpy road for EBM in this non-clinical area of decision making. Two of these examples relate to screening for different types of cancer and the third to decision making related to the integration of CAM.

EBM on a Bumpy Road in Political Decision Making: Three Examples

Example 1: The Case of Breast Cancer Screening

The first example considered here is screening for breast cancer. Decisions about screening generally take place on a national level, driven by groups of experts in the specific field of medicine. Screening, within this context, is the search for non-symptomatic disease in a population (Holland, Stewart and Masseria 2006) and may include the testing of asymptomatic individuals. Screening with mammography uses x-ray in order to identify breast tumours before they can be felt in a physical examination. The goal is to treat breast cancer earlier when a cure is more likely (Gøtzsche and Nielsen 2009). Screening for breast cancer is most commonly offered to women between the ages of 50–69 with the greatest benefit shown in women aged 60–69 years (United States Preventive Services Task Force 2009).

The introduction of screening programmes for breast cancer, however, has been controversial and has been described as a key challenge for evidence-based models of healthcare delivery (Goodman 2002). Research, for example, has recently seriously questioned the efficacy of breast cancer screening in reducing mortality (Gøtzsche and Nielsen 2009, Jørgensen, Zahl and Gøtzsche 2010). At the core of this debate are methodological concerns about bias, deficient meta-analyses and weakness of trials that indicate benefit (Gøtzsche and Nielsen 2009). Furthermore, due to the almost exclusive focus on early diagnosis, there is a realthreat of false positive findings, resulting in significant harm for women receiving unnecessary intervention (Gøtzsche and Nielsen 2009). Such harm includes psychological distress, unnecessary imaging tests and biopsies in women without cancer and inconvenience due to false-positive screening results (United States Preventive Services Task Force 2009). Despite this, currently, screening for breast cancer in women aged 50–69 years is not a subject of considerable debate outside the confines of this particular medical sub-specialty and research community.

The debate surrounding breast cancer screening for the 40–49 age group however, is more heated and has entered the political and public sphere. Research indicates that if 3,000 women aged 40 years are not screened for breast cancer, 2,922 women will be alive after 13 years. If they are screened, 2,923 women will survive. Over the same time period, ten women will be diagnosed with a precursor of cancer that does not develop into cancer (Norwegian Knowledge Centre for Health Services 2007). Although Governments do tend to acknowledge these figures, internationally varying political decisions have been made regarding screening in the 40–49 age group. In Australia, for example, recruitment strategies for screening are targeted at women aged 50–69, although women above 40 are eligible. This means that women in this lower age group can choose to be screened but are not specifically targeted. Australian authorities have for the time being concluded that 'current evidence indicated that the benefits of breast cancer screening for women aged 40–49 years are not strong enough to encourage all women in this age group to have regular breast cancer screening', but that they are able to have a free screening mammogram if they wish (Breastscreen Victoria 2010).

In Norway screening is not offered as a free service to women aged 40–49 years. The question as to whether they should was reconsidered in a report written by the Norwegian Knowledge Centre for the Health Services in 2007 but screening was not recommended or implemented (The Directorate for Health and Social Affairs 2007). This was due to studies that indicated the burdensome effects of false positives among other negative outcomes (Norwegian Knowledge Centre for Health Services 2007). In the US, on the other hand, the Preventive Task Force recommended screening for American women aged 40–49 in 2002 (United States Preventive Services Task Force 2002), emphasising that for many women 'the potential reduction in risk for death due to breast cancer associated with screening will outweigh other considerations' (United States Preventive Services Task Force 2002: 514). Such differences illustrate the political embeddedness and differential utilisation of 'evidence' internationally. Moreover, such varying forms of screening policy illustrate how ideas about choice, the cultural 'protection' of women, and cultures of risk (or risk avoidance) shape a government's willingness to utilise of evidence on a national scale.

The political character of decision about breast cancer screening – rather than its evidence-base – was illustrated in November 2009 when the US Preventive Task Force removed its recommendations for screening women aged 40–49. This move reflected the perspective that regular biennial screening mammography before the age of 50 years should be an individual decision (United States Preventive Services Task Force 2009). However, when these new recommendations were released in November 2009, the White House backed away from implementing them (Furlow 2010) and the issue appears to be unresolved at time of publication. In this case at least, it points to the bumpy road for evidence-based medicine in terms of the tensions between what 'works empirically' and 'what is acceptable politically'. Reviewing the debate so far, John McKinlay (2009) argues that 'the success or failure of clinical guidelines is presently determined by political process' (McKinlay 2009: 5).

Further support of the unpredictable and bumpy road argument for EBM is available from the Norwegian experience of the introduction of mammographic screening. In Norway, breast cancer screening was piloted in four counties from 1996. However, politicians in Norway did not await evaluations from the initial project of mammography screening in the four counties before deciding upon a nationwide screening programme (Solbjør 2008), illustrating the tense balance between political decisions and evidence-based decisions.

Example 2: Prostate Cancer Screening

Until the invention of the Prostate Specific Antigen (PSA) test in 1970, the standard means of screening for prostate cancer was the Digital Rectal Examination (DRE). The PSA was originally discovered by Richard Ablin as a means of tracking the presence and progress in size of a prostate tumour (Ablin 2010). The actual PSA test appears to have been developed by Ming Chua at the Roswell Park Cancer Institute, to whom a patent was issued in 1984 (Mohler 2010). At first the test received Food and Drug Administration (FDA) approval in 1986 only to monitor treatment response and disease recurrence. Only later in 1994, when the global market for screening for diagnosis became apparent, did the FDA approve its use for this purpose (Mohler 2010).

Once the wider potential for the PSA test was recognised, demand soared given it was a non-invasive alternative to Digital Rectal Examination. A profit-driven technological imperative operated with surge in usage of PSA technology, advocated and promoted by men's groups, fuelled by stories of men who would no longer be alive but for the timely PSA intervention. By 2010, Albin (2010) stated that in the US alone, some 30 million men underwent testing at a cost of US$3 billion annually. Yet, from the outset of the career of PSA screening as a medical technology, questions about efficacy and cost surfaced and many countries established health technology assessment inquiries. EW was a member of the Australian inquiry (AHTAC 1996) and published a sociological analysis of the debate and subsequent policy decisions (Willis 1997). Although the inquiry was assisted in their deliberations by biomedical 'evidence', this late 1990s period was one where EBM was being codified as a health technology by various advocates (e.g. Sackett et al. 1996). Even then, the ability of the inquiry to definitively answer the question of whether population screening was safe, efficacious and cost effective was hampered by the ongoing randomised trials being carried out simultaneously in the US and Europe. The state of knowledge at the time was that the benefit of screening with PSA (or DRE for that matter) was unknown. At the time there had been no comprehensive analysis of the trade-off between risks and benefits.

A decade later these two trials have both reported their results. While their meaning is being digested and debated in medical circles they do appear, at very least, to undermine the evidence base for PSA screening technology. The US trial (Andriole et al. 2009) showed that over a period of seven to ten years, screening did not reduce mortality from prostate cancer in men aged 55 years and over. The European study (Schröder et al. 2009) did show a small decline in death rates but also found that 48 men would need to be treated to save one man's life. In the light of these findings some prestigious medical bodies have changed their recommendations. The American College of Preventive Medicine now recommends against routine screening citing insufficient evidence (Ablin 2010). In a decision Ablin describes as 'shameful', the American Urological Association still recommends screening while other eminent bodies such as the National Cancer Institute and the American Cancer Society are more equivocal and vague, arguing that the evidence is still not clear (Ablin 2010).

The appearance of the opinion piece in the *New York Times* by the original discoverer of the PSA, Richard Ablin (2010), arguably marks a move to the stage of 'denunciation' (McKinlay 1981: 395–6) in the debate on PSA. In a strongly worded attack on the continued use of PSA as a screening tool, Ablin argues that the test is hardly more effective than a coin toss; it cannot actually do what it promises which is to detect prostate cancer, nor can it distinguish between the lethal and non-lethal types of malignancies. While he argues that PSA testing does retain its original usage in marking the course of the disease and for men with a family history, he concludes:

> I never dreamed that my discovery four decades ago would lead to such a profit driven public health disaster. The medical community must confront reality and stop the inappropriate use of PSA screening. Doing so would save billions of dollars and rescue millions of men from unnecessary, debilitating treatments. (Ablin 2010)

Example 3: EBM and the Integration of CAM

The last example we present draws on the process the integration of CAM modalities in health care. Integration of CAM modalities has become an issue in health care particularly during the last decade. This is due to an assumed change in health care within western populations, in which health care users orient themselves towards and use a broader range of health care services, and in which the previously held superior position of a biomedical approach to health and illness is increasingly challenged (Coulter and Willis 2004). Some have gone as far as suggesting that we are witnessing the rise of an integrative medicine, in which biomedicine and CAM are combined (Baer and Coulter 2008).

The integration of CAM into conventional health care, however, is problematised when it is assessed according to the central tenets of evidence-based health care. The evidence (at least within the accepted frame for scientific evidence that operates in western health care) on the effects of CAM modalities is patchy and high level biomedical evidence for many modalities/practices is scarce. This has presented a barrier to CAM integration in many clinical contexts. The current situation is that few CAM treatments are implemented in terms of prompting financial coverage by the public health care system (see, for example, McCabe 2005). There are requests for more research that can strengthen the evidence-base for CAM (in conventional terms) while researchers in the CAM field experience difficulties in securing such research funding (Coulter and Willis 2004). Independent of what appears as the most relevant explanation on the lack of an evidence-base, the process of integrating CAM modalities in health care appears to be framed by the current standards of what counts as 'evidence-based'.

As with the previous examples, however, there is not a straightforward, unproblematic implementation of EBM type findings in addressing issues related to CAM integration with conventional medicine. Instead there is a more complex implementation process involved. This is illustrated by an example from Norway and relates to the health information that the health care system provides the population. The example comes from what can be considered the 'fringe' of health care and is at a clear distance from core clinical work and decisions about screening programs. Nevertheless, it is still important as an illustration of the range of processes in which EBM plays a role.

The example we present concerns the establishment of an information centre for CAM that was opened in 2008 and run by the Norwegian Government called the 'National Information Center for Complementary and Alternative Medicine, Norway' (NIFAB). NIFAB is a public information centre for alternative treatment affiliated with the National Research Centre in Complementary and Alternative Medicine (NAFKAM) at the University of Tromsoe. NIFAB aims to help consumers make informed choices in their health care. Provision of information is part of public health care and takes place within the requirements of evidence-based health care. The decision to establish this information centre was taken in 2006 as a result of increased use of CAM. The government emphasised a need to provide balanced information because of the range of commercial interests involved in CAM and the potential for health care users to be exposed to flawed information (The Ministry of Health Norway 2005). In February 2009, the centre advertised that it exists to provide information which is not rooted in any particular explanation model of health and illness (Gundersen, Sundby and Storm 2009).

The establishment of this centre has not been without contestation. In February 2009, 15 medical doctors and biologists signed a letter to the Norwegian Ministry of Health, in which they questioned the funding of NIFAB and proposed that the centre should be phased out. They presented a critical assessment of the information provided at NIFAB's website, arguing that NIFAB avoids including scientific studies in the information that is provided (author's translation) and that the content on the website is mainly based on information provided by CAM organisations (Gundersen, Sundby and Storm 2009). The Ministry of Health asked for a response, which was provided by the Medical Faculty at the University of

Tromsoe, NAFKAM and NIFAB at the end of March in the same year (Straume, Fønnebø and Lillenes 2009). The response acknowledged that a scientific view on different CAM treatments should be more visible, while defending the activity at the centre. NIFAB has continued to receive funding in 2010 (The Ministry of Health Norway 2009), although the statement about the need to provide information that is not rooted in 'any particular explanation model of health and illness' was removed from the website.

The Future Research Agenda

This final section provides an outline for a future research agenda for social science research on EBHC. It underscores the need to look beyond the broader implementation of EBM, EBP and their various manifestations, and to consider in more detail the clinical context and political decision-making processes. The questions raised in relation to the third example above are given particular attention, but the discussion starts by offering some reflections related to the clinical context, which adds to a growing body of literature focusing on this issue (Broom, Adams and Tovey 2009, Knaapen et al. 2010, Moreira 2005, Mykhalovskiy and Weir 2004, Timmermans and Mauck 2005).

The Clinical Context: Situational and Local Frames

The introductory part of this chapter provided a picture of the clinical context in which the impact of CPGs is demonstrated as highly variable (Carlsen, Glenton and Pope 2007, McKinlay et al. 2004, Timmermans and Almeling 2009, Timmermans and Mauck 2005). In their contribution, Timmermans and Mauck (2005) argue that the success of the current EBM paradigm has been constrained by its orientation toward a traditional image of the autonomous medical profession decision maker. These authors suggest that the collaborative nature of medical work needs to be taken into consideration when implementing evidence-based medicine. Timmermans and Mauck direct attention to the organisation of clinical care and the need for a more detailed understanding of the context of EBM implementation. A further question that can be raised is the impact of team environments on such processes. A call for more research on this issue is timely given that multidisciplinary work in health care is widespread.

When it comes to production of clinical practical guidelines more knowledge is needed. Guideline development can be an unpredictable process and there are few studies that address development processes from a critical social science perspective (Knaapen et al. 2010). Those who have explored guideline development point to the professional status of those involved (Pagliari and Grimshaw 2002) and that a situational impact takes place (Knaapen et al. 2010, Moreira 2005). A more thorough understanding of such processes will not solve conflicts that emerge in relation to guideline development, such as the disagreementsoutlined above in the context of breast cancer screening. What it will do is contribute to the conceptualisation of the complexity of such processes. Among the potential implications is an increased impact of CPGs in practice. As Moreira (2005) argues, by attending to the diversity of forms of knowledge at work in guideline development, guideline committees can 'construct knowledge that takes into consideration the diverse worlds in which the guidelines can be used' (Moreira 2005: 1984)

The role and centrality of RCTs and other epidemiological designs strategies is a core issue when it comes to guideline development. Although there is widespread agreement that RCTs are the gold standard (in the context of interventions) and of crucial importance in guideline development, there are large areas of medicine that are not open to evaluation by experimental designs (Lambert, Gordon and Bogdon-Lovis 2006, Grootendorst et al. 2010). In some situations it might be unnecessary, inappropriate, impossible or inadequate to run an RCT (Grootendorst et al. 2010). Moreover, as commented by Lambert, Gordon and Bogdon-Lovis (2006), patients' views on what works can differ from those of researchers and practitioners. This can create tensions when attempts are made to combine, or balance, evidence-based approaches to health care with the views and preferences of patients receiving health care. On the other hand though, more attention is currently being paid to the applicability of RCTs, as demonstrated for example by the study conducted by Grootendorst et al. (2010). Such attention contributes to an assessment of one of the important elements in guideline development and decision making in health care more generally.

Political Decision Making: The Need to Explore Patient Perspectives and Account for Context-Dependent Decision Processes

The argument in this chapter is that the success of EBM implementation and evidence-based health care more broadly should not be taken for granted. That is, it is increasingly evident that 'evidence' is politically shaped/implemented (i.e. in the case of screening), and moreover, evidence-based models are being utilised as a form of reductive inter-professional power (i.e. in relation to CAM integration). These cases, and the others examined in this book, provide an important reminder of the importance of utilising the resources of the social sciences to offer critical and nuanced analyses of evidence-based models *in practice*.

One potential area of further inquiry is the 'patient perspective' that underpins the concerns many social scientists have about the consequences of EBHC. Such concerns are embedded in an assumed incongruence between biomedical approaches and people's individual experiences of health and illness (see, for example, Conrad 2005). Yet, this assumption of distance or disconnect has also been questioned in terms of whether biomedical conceptions can 'provide an objective fixed point on a terrain of uncertainty' (Bury 1982: 179; see also Bishop and Yardley 2004; Sandaunet 2008). This work has illustrated the importance of not taking for granted the ontological distance between people/patients and the proponents of EBHC. In terms of CAM integration, this underscores the need for an open minded exploration of how this example of 'EBM at work' corresponds to individual experiences, including the possibility that EBHC-type models might validate patient perspectives.

In saying this, the national contexts in which political decisions are made need to be better understood. For example, the debate on the effects of breast cancer screening demonstrate that, while the implementation of EBM takes place in a seemingly shared 'western context' of health delivery and is based on a common source of evidence, the implementation of EBM in different cultural contexts is actually highly differentiated. Political decision-making processes are made not only to ensure effectiveness, but also aimed at maximising what has come to be called patient-centred health care. At the core of the breast cancer screening debate is the issue of the harm provided by screening, in contrast to the potential prevention of the development of a serious illness. This appears to be viewed quite differentially depending on the given national context. The issue hinges around conceptualising what patient-centred health care actually means. Both the aim of reducing mortality and avoiding harm do, ultimately, seek to ensure patient-centred health care. Yet these arguments seem to be given different emphasis in different national contexts. One clear method of exploring how *person-centred* these different approaches are is embarking on further examination, across different cultures, of patient perspectives and values in and around the importance of forms of knowledge, relative risk and harm.

Individual accounts of care (and the role of forms of evidence therein) would provide an important contrast to the cultural and political idiosyncrasies in health delivery. In Europe, health technology assessments have tended to pay more attention to broader social implications, especially issues such as ethics and threats to solidarity (Banta 2003). In Norway, as we have indicated, unnecessary harm is more significant within decision making about breast screening whereas in the (litigious, risk-averse US) the choice not to screen is a much more 'prevent at all costs' dynamic. Such scenarios remind us that political decision making inevitably involves value judgments (Shaw and Greenhalgh 2008, Sanderson 2006) whereas evidence-based models are (theoretically) underpinned by an instrumental rationality that attempts to minimise ethical and moral considerations (Sanderson 2006). A conflict of this type was evident in the continued funding for an information centre for complementary and alternative medicine in Norway as a public's right *vis-à-vis* an appropriate 'evidence base'. Inevitably, political decision making that concerns health issues, for example related to CAM, must account both for requirements consideration of therapeutic legitimacy *and* person-oriented care. Within this frame, the intentions of CAM integration, such as providing information about CAM treatments, can be argued to lack a 'scientific' basis, but may still be relevant within the contemporary image of person-oriented health care.

The conventional tools for supporting political decision making are Health Technology Assessment (HTA) and Comparative Effectiveness Research (CER). The discussion above suggests the need to rethink the question of how far both the evidence and associated HTA/CER methodologies assist politicians in their decisions. In fact, it is clear that EBHC often has limited impact on policy making, and even techniques designed to consider multiple factors in introducing forms of care, including HTA, have been consistently influenced by policy-makers concerns about expenditures (Banta 2003). While Banta points to a difference between the US and Europe with respect to the emphasis placed on social and ethical issues, he points to the influence of considerations about expenditures in both (see also May 2006: 528–9).

CER requires further exploration as an evaluation tool taking into account value judgements and legal considerations in decision making (Chalkidou et al. 2009) as well as reducing reliance on RCT's for evidence of effectiveness (Chalkidou et al. 2009, Coulter 2011). Coulter (2011) provides an interesting contribution to this literature. He analyses the initiative in the US towards emphasising Comparative Effectiveness Research (CER) and the consequences for the CAM area. Welcomed by many CAM researchers, CER allows recognition of new or previously unacknowledged forms of evidence, focusing on the outcomes of treatment, not the underlying explanations for why they work (Coulter and Willis 2007). This has had significant advantages, for example, for chiropractic. No longer would the chiropractic community have to demonstrate the assumptive bases underpinning why spinal manipulation is effective; just that it is (Shekelle et al. 1992). Coulter (2011), adopting a critical social science perspective, still asks whether the evolution of CER may just be a new form of privileging certain forms of evidence and knowledge at the expense of other equally important, and perhaps more relevant, forms. He warns that it is possible that a reliance on CER in the United States might also perpetuate a powerful ideology that could be used against CAM. In sum, further research is needed to explore the implications of HTA and CER and how they may assist and influence policy making processes.

Conclusion

The aim of this concluding chapter has been to outline a future research agenda for social science research on EBM. In a purely rational world, one would expect the process of EBM implementation to be rather straightforward. Demonstrated evidence from well-designed methods of evaluation would lead to changes in clinical practice. In many instances this is the case. Yet the translation of evidence into practice is far from straightforward and apolitical, as demonstrated in this chapter and this book as a whole. This final chapter has utilised the metaphor of a 'bumpy road' for EBM to make suggestions for further research on evidence-based health care. In particular, the need to explore the impact of local and situational factors on EBM implementation. Moreover, to assess the use and relevance of clinical practice guidelines in multidisciplinary settings or the relations between 'evidence' and political decision making in different national contexts. Finally, to systematically document and integrate patient perspectives within a range of clinical contexts and to map their correspondence with the current manifestations of evidence-based health care. Critically documenting the localised, political and subjective aspects of knowledge production and implementation would provide much needed insight into how EBHC is shaping healthcare delivery in the twenty-first century. This book provides only a glimpse into the social world of EBHC in context and there remains a large number of areas that would benefit from the application of a critical social science perspective.

References

Ablin, R. 2010. *The Great Prostate Mistake.* [Online]. *New York Times.* Available at: www.nytimes.com/2010/3/10opinion/10Ablin.html [accessed: 14 January 2011].

Andriole, G., Crawford, E., Grubb, R., Buys, S., Chia, D., Church, T., Fouad, M., Gelmann, E., Kvale, P., Reding, D., Weissfeld, J., Yokochi, L., O'Brien, B., Clapp, J., Rathmell, J., Riley, T., Hayes, R., Kramer, B., Izmirlian, G., Anthony, B., Pinsky, P., Prorok, P., Gohagan, J. and Berg, C. 2009. Mortality results from a randomized prostate-cancer screening trial. *New England Journal of Medicine*, 360(13), 1310–19.

Baer, H. and Coulter, I. 2008. Introduction: Taking stock of integrative medicine: Broadening biomedicine or co-option of complementary and alternative medicine? *Health Sociology Review*, 17(4), 331–41.

Banta, D. 2003. The development of health technology assessment. *Health Policy*, 63(2), 121–32.

Behague, D., Tawiah, C., Rosato, M., Some, T. and Morrison, J. 2009. Evidence-based policy-making: The implications of globally-applicable research for context-specific problem-solving in developing countries. *Social Science and Medicine*, 69(10), 1539–46.

Bishop, F. and Yardley, L. 2004. Constructing agency in treatment decisions: Negotiating responsibility in cancer. *Health: An Interdisciplinary Journal for the Social Study of Health, Illness and Medicine*, 8(4), 465–82.

Breastscreen Victoria. 2010. *About Screening.* [Online: Breastscreen Victoria]. Available at: www.breastscreen.org.au/index.php?option=com_content&task=view&id=4&Itemid=5 [accessed: 20 March 2010].

Broom, A., Adams, J. and Tovey, P. 2009. Evidence-based healthcare in practice: A study of clinician resistance, professional de-skilling and inter-specialty differentiation in oncology. *Social Science and Medicine*, 68(1), 192–200.

Bury, M. 1982. Chronic illness as biographical disruption. *Sociology of Health and Illness*, 4(2), 167–82.

Carlsen, B., Glenton, C. and Pope, B. 2007. Thou shalt versus thou shalt not: A meta-synthesis of GP's attitudes to clinical practical guidelines. *British Journal of General Practice*, 57(545), 971–8.

Chalkidou, K., Tunis, S., Lopert, R., Rochaix, L., Sawicki, P., Nasser, M. and Xerri, B. 2009. Comparative effectiveness research and evidence-based health policy: Experience from four countries. *The Milbank Quarterly*, 87(2), 339–67.

Conrad, P. 2005. *The Sociology of Health and Illness, Critical Perpectives.* New York: Worth Publishers.

Coulter, A. and Magee, H. 2003. *The European Patient of the Future.* Maidenhead: Open University Press.

Coulter, I. 2011. Comparative effectiveness research: Does the emperor have clothes? *Alternative Therapies in Health and Medicine*, 17(2), 8–15.

Coulter, I. and Willis, E. 2004. The rise and rise of complementary and alternative medicine: A sociological perspective. *The Medical Journal of Australia*, 180(11), 587–9.

Coulter, I. and Willis, E. 2007. Explaining the growth of complementary and alternative medicine. *Health Sociology Review*, 16(3–4), 214–25.

Field, M. and Lohr, K. 1990. *Clinical Practical Guidelines: Directions for a New Program.* Washington, DC: National Academic Press.

Frankford, D. 1994. Scientism and economics in the regulation of health care. *Journal of Health Politics, Policy and Law*, 19(4), 773–99.

Furlow, B. 2010. US evidence-based medicine faces uphill battle. *The Lancet Oncology*, 11(1), 15.

Goodman, S. 2002. The mammography dilemma: A crisis for evidence-based medicine. *Annals of Internal Medicine*, 137(5), 363–5.

Grootendorst, D., Jager, K., Zocalli, C. and Dekker, F. 2010. Observational studies are complementary to randomized controlled trials. *Nephron Clinical Practice*, 114(3), 173–7.

Gundersen, K., Sundby, I. and Storm, J. 2009. The activities at the National Information Center for Complementary and Alternative Treatment, Norway. *Letter to the Ministry of Health and Care Services, Norway.* [Online]. Available at: www.fritanke.no/filarkiv/03_kritikk_av_nifab.pdf [accessed: 20 April 2011].

Gøtzsche, P. and Nielsen, M. 2009. Screening for breast cancer with mammography (Review). *The Cochrane Database of Systematic Reviews*, October 7; (4): CD001877.

Hoggan, J. and Littlemore, R. 2009. *Climate Cover-Up: The Crusade to Deny Global Warning.* Vancouver: Greystone Books.

Holland, W., Stewart, S. and Masseria, C. 2006. *Screening in Europe.* Policy Brief. [Online: The European Observatory on Health Systems and Policies]. Available at: www.euro.int/_data/assets/pdf_file/0007/108961/E88698.pdf [accessed: 20 April 2011].

Jørgensen, K., Zahl, P. and Gøtzsche, P. 2010. Breast cancer mortality in organised mammography screening in Denmark: Comparative study. *British Medical Journal*, 340: c1241.

Knaapen, L., Cazeneuve, H., Cambrosio, A., Castel, P. and Fervers, B. 2010. Pragmatic evidence and textual arrangements: A case study of French clinical cancer guidelines. *Social Science and Medicine*, 71(4), 685–92.

Lambert, H., Gordon, E. and Bogdan-Lovis, E. 2006. Introduction: Gift horse or trojan horse? Social science perspectives on evidence-based health care. *Social Science and Medicine*, 62(11), 2613–20.

May, C. 2006. Mobilising modern facts: Health technology assessment and the politics of evidence. *Sociology of Health and Illness*, 28(5), 513–32.

McCabe, P. 2005. Complementary and alternative medicine in Australia: A contemporary overview. *Complementary Therapies in Clinical Practice*, 11(1), 28–31.

McKinlay, E., McLeod, D., Dowell, A. and Marshall, C. 2004. Clinical practice guidelines' development and use in New Zealand: an evolving process. *The New Zealand Medical Journal*, 117(1199). [Online]. Available at: http://www.nzma.org.nz/journal/117-1199/999/ [accessed: 20 April 2011].

McKinlay, J. 1981. From 'promising report' to 'standard procedure': Seven stages in the stages in the career of a medical innovation. *The Milbank Memorial Fund Quarterly: Health and Society*, 59(3), 374–411.

McKinlay, J. 2009. The Mammo Controversy – So much for evidence-based medicine. *News and Views*. [Online: New England Research Institutes]. Available at: www.neriscience.com/Portals/0/Uploads/Documents/Public/Mammo_Controversy.pdf [accessed: 20 April 2011].

Mohler, J. 2010. *PSA and the PSA Test: What the Public Needs to Know*. [Online: Roswell Park Cancer Institute, New York]. Available at: http://www.roswellpark.org/media/news/psa-and-psa-test-what-public-needs-know [accessed: 7 April 2010].

Moreira, T. 2005. Diversity in clinical guidelines: The role of repertoires of evaluation. *Social Science and Medicine*, 60(9), 1975–85.

Mykhalovskiy, E. and Weir, L. 2004. The problem of evidence-based medicine: Directions for social science. *Social Science and Medicine*, 59(5), 1059–69.

Norwegian Knowledge Centre for Health Services. 2007. Mammography screening of women 40–49. *Report*, Issue 9. [Online: Norwegian Knowledge Centre for Health Services]. Available at: www.kunnskapssenteret.no/Publikasjoner/Mammografiscreening+av+kvinner+40%E2%80%9349+%C3%A5r.864.cms?language=english [accessed: 20 April 2011].

Pagliari, C. and Grimshaw, J. 2002. Impact of group structure and process on multidisciplinary evidence-based guideline development: An observational study. *Journal of Evaluation in Clinical Practice*, 8(2), 145–53.

Pope, C. 2003. Resisting evidence: The study of evidence-based medicine as a contemporary social movement. *Health: An Interdisciplinary Journal for the Social Study of Health, Illness and Medicine*, 7(3), 267–82.

Rodwin, M. 2001. The politics of evidence-based medicine. *Journal of Health Politics, Policy and Law*, 26(2), 439–45.

Sackett, D., Rosenberg, W., Gray, J., Haynes, R. and Richardson, W. 1996. Evidence based medicine: What it is and what it isn't. *British Medical Journal*, 312(7023), 71–2.

Sandaunet, A. 2008. The challenge of fitting in: Non-participation and withdrawal from an online self-help group for Norwegian breast cancer patients. *Sociology of Health and Illness*, 30(1), 131–44.

Sanderson, I. 2006. Complexity, 'practical rationality' and evidence based policy making. *Policy and Politics*, 34(1), 115–32.

Schröder, F., Hugosson, J., Roobol, M., Tammela, T., Ciatto, S., Nelen, V., Kwiatkowski, M., Lujan, M., Lilja, H., Zappa, M., Denis, L., Recker, F., Berenguer, A., Määttänen, L., Bangma, C., Aus, G., Villers, A., Rebillard, X., van der Kwast, T., Blijenberg, B., Moss, S., de Koning, H. and Auvinen, A. 2009. Screening and prostate-cancer mortality in a randomized European study. *New England Journal of Medicine*, 360, 1320–28.

Shaneyfelt, T. and Centor, R. 2009. Reassessment of clinical practical guidelines: Go gently into that night. *Journal of the American Medical Association*, 301(8), 868–9.

Shaw, S. and Greenhalgh, T. 2008. Best research – for what? Best health – for whom? A critical exploration of primary care research using discourse analysis. *Social Science and Medicine*, 66(12), 2506–19.

Shekelle, P., Adams, A., Chassin, M., Hurwitz, E. and Brook, R. 1992. Spinal manipulation for low-back pain. *Annals of Internal Medicine*, 117(7), 590–98.

Solbjør, M. 2008. Women's experience of mammography screening: Decision making, participation and recall. *Doctoral Thesis.* [Online: Faculty of Social Sciences and Technology Management. Trondheim, Norwegian University of Science and Technology]. Available at: urn.kb.se/resolve?urn=urn:nbn:no:ntn u:diva-2330 [accessed: 20 April 2011].

Straume, B.J., Fønnebø, V. and Lillenes, O. (2009). Response to letter concerning the activity at NIFAB – the National Information Center for Complementary and Alternative Treatment, Norway. *Letter to the Ministry of Health and Care Services, Norway.* [Online]. Available at: www.fritanke.no/filarkiv/04_svar_ fra_nifab.pdf [accessed: 20 April 2011].

The Directorate for Health and Social Affairs. 2007. National action plan with guidelines for diagnosis, treatment and follow-up for patients with breast cancer 2006–2009. *National Guidelines.* [Online: The Directorate of Health, Norway]. Available at: www.shdir.no/vp/multimedia/archive/00021/ Nasjonalt_handlingsp_21559a.pdf [accessed: 20 April 2011].

The Ministry of Health Norway. 2005. *Parliamentary Bill*, Issue 1 (2005–2006). [Online: The Ministry of Health Norway]. Available at: www.regjeringen.no/ Rpub/STP/20052006/001HOD/PDFS/STP200520060001HODDDDPDFS. pdf [accessed: 20 April 2011].

The Ministry of Health Norway. 2009. *Parliamentary Bill*, Issue 1 (2009–2010). [Online: The Ministry of Health Norway]. Available at: www.regjeringen.no/pages/2250451/PDFS/PRP200920100001HODDDDPDFS.pdf [accessed: 20 April 2011].

Timmermans, S. and Almeling, R. 2009. Objectification, standardization, and commodification in health care: A conceptual readjustment. *Social Science and Medicine*, 69(1), 21–7.

Timmermans, S. and Berg, M. 2003. *The Gold Standard: A Challenge of Evidence-Based Medicine and Standardisation of Health Care.* Philadelphia: Temple University Press.

Timmermans, S. and Mauck, A. 2005. The promises and pitfalls of evidence-based medicine. *Health Affairs*, 24(1), 18–27.

US Preventive Services Task Force. 2002. Screening for breast cancer: Recommendations and rationale. *Annals of Internal Medicine*, 137(5), 344–6.

US Preventive Services Task Force. 2008. Grade Definitions. May 2008. [Online: US Preventive Task Force]. Available at: www.uspreventiveservicestaskforce.org/uspstf/grades.htm.

US Preventive Services Task Force. 2009. Screening for breast cancer: US Preventive Task Forces recommendation statement. *Annals of Internal Medicine*, 151(10), 716–26.

Willis, E. 1997. The prostate initiative and the social relations of medical technology. *International Journal of Technology Assessment in Health Care*, 13(4), 602–12.

Index